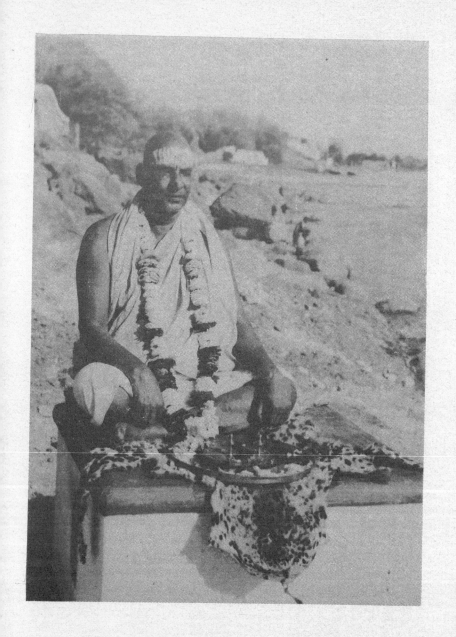

H.H. SWAMI SIVANANDAJI MAHARAJ

# PRACTICAL LESSONS IN YOGA

*Swami Sivananda*

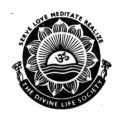

*Published By*

THE DIVINE LIFE SOCIETY
P.O. SHIVANANDANAGAR—249 192
Distt. Tehri-Garhwal, U.P., Himalayas, India

Price ]                    1997                    [ Rs. 60/-

Eighth Edition: 1997
(6,000 Copies)

Published by Swami Krishnananda for The Divine Life
Society, Shivanandanagar, and printed by him
at the Yoga-Vedanta Forest Academy Press,
P.O. Shivanandanagar, Distt. Tehri-Garhwal,
U.P., Himalayas, India

TO
STUDENTS OF YOGA
IN
**THE EAST AND THE WEST**

# PUBLISHERS' NOTE

His Holiness Sri Swami Sivananda Saraswati is, as it were, an ornament of not only the glorious Himalayas and India but of the entire world. From the cool heights of his Himalayan Ashram, "Ananda Kutir," the great Yogi stood as a mighty dynamo radiating Divine Love, Joy and Peace to millions upon millions of bleeding hearts all over the world, a Yogi, who shines as a brilliant pole-star in the spiritual firmament of the universe, guiding the tired and restless traveller towards the haven of Peace, Bliss and Knowledge.

As a great saint and philosopher, his spotless purity, saintliness of life, magnetic and voluminous writings were unparalleled in record; he was not only an eminent and popular author of Hindu religious and philosophical subjects, but is an authority on those subjects. He was not only a man of letters and vast erudition, but also one who had in a full measure realised the incalculable benefits of Yogic practices in the course of a strenuous struggle of over fifteen years of intense dispassion and rigorous austerities in the holy regions of the Himalayas. Moreover, his priceless writings through the medium of some of the well-known and influential newspapers, magazines and journals not only in India but also abroad and in America coupled with his own unique and powerful personality and realisation have won for him an enviable place of honour in every spiritually, religiously and philosophically inclined home in India. In fact, if the political India of the present

v

day can be proud of at least one Gandhi, the spiritual India can be reasonably proud of at least one Sivananda!

The object with which this book is published is twofold. Year in and year out large numbers of Europeans and Americans, men and women, came out to India to learn Yoga under an Adept and practise the same in India itself. In the course of their endless wanderings and searches for such Adepts in Yoga, these people had no other alternative but to resort to the Himalayan Ashram of Swami Sivananda. But unfortunately owing to several causes these travellers could not remain long in this country. They went back home learning something here and something there, in bits, but nothing from one Yogi only, which alone could be said to be of some solid and practical utility to them.

The Westerners, interested in Yogic practices, had naturally to take resort to books and other literature on the subject, which were either unintelligible to them or, as was more often than not, had been written by persons whose aim in writing books was, in ninety-nine cases out of every hundred, to show off their learning rather than to teach Yoga and make the subject intelligible and interesting to the public. This is the difference between books written by most writers and those by Swami Sivananda. Moreover, unlike several others, Swami Sivananda Saraswati was a practical Yogi, who fully realised the fruits of Yoga and was therefore best suited to write books on the subject from his own practical experience. The present book has been specially designed by the author keeping in mind the needs of the students of Yoga in Europe and America, who need a practical but non-technical presentation of the subject in a language which is accessible to the beginner in the path. We hope the book will amply serve this most sacred purpose in view.

May the unfailing blessings of Swami Sivananda pour forth in profusion over the heads of all the readers in the West and East, nay, North and South, and lead them on to *Satchidananda*, which every one is seeking at heart!

THE DIVINE LIFE SOCIETY

# PREFACE

This book entitled "Practical Lessons in Yoga" consists of twelve easy and interesting Lessons. The First Lesson deals with Yoga and Its Objects. The Second Lesson treats of Yoga Sadhana or the practice of Yoga and contains a clear and lucid description of the four important paths viz., Karma Yoga, Bhakti Yoga, Raja Yoga and Jnana Yoga. One can easily choose for himself a path according to his particular taste, temperament and capacity by a close study of this Lesson. I firmly hold that no one wishing to become a perfect Yogi can realise his wish, if he does not begin his Yogic practices with Karma Yoga or doing actions for actions' sake, without the idea of agency and without expectation of the fruits of his actions. I have also made passing references to the various other forms of Yoga such as Hatha Yoga, Mantra Yoga and Kundalini Yoga.

In the Third Lesson on Yogic Discipline I have clearly and expressly stated that the practice of Yoga is rooted in the cultivation of virtues and the eradication of negative qualities, and have also stated in detail what virtues should of necessity be cultivated and what vices are to be eradicated, and through what means.

Yogic Diet forms the subject-matter of the Fourth Lesson. It should be distinctly borne in mind that mind is made up of the fine particles of food that we take, and we are what we eat. If the student of Yoga who is a neophyte desires to lay a firm, sure and sound foundation in his

viii

practices, he should take care to eat only such foods that are conducive to his spiritual advancement and progress, and avoid all others. A list of the various articles of diet, prescribed and prohibited, is also given.

In the Fifth Lesson I have taken all care to collect the various stumbling blocks in the way of the aspirant and the various means of overcoming them. I strongly advise the student to read and re-read this Lesson a number of times in order that he may be cautious in moments of temptation.

Then in the Sixth Lesson I have dealt with Yogasanas or Yogic postures. It is very necessary for the would-be Yogi to maintain a sound and vigorous body and mind to achieve success in his undertaking, and in order that he might achieve this end, a number of simple and easy exercises, physical and consequently mental, have been prescribed. These exercises were practised by Yogins and Rishis of yore and are still being practised in India and other countries with astonishing results.

The Seventh Lesson treats of Pranayama or regulation of breath. Simple and practical exercises have been prescribed for the regulation and control of breath, which will ultimately result in the control of the mind. These exercises in breath-control are not merely for enhancing the soundness and control of the mind, but they also play a vital part in ensuring a sound body. The student of Pranayama, who attains perfection in it, will have various psychic powers.

Regulation of breath and control of mind lead to concentration. So concentration is the topic of the next lesson. I have dealt at length with the nature of the mind and the methods through which it can be controlled. Some practical exercises are given to attain success in concentration.

The Ninth Lesson deals with Meditation because the fruit of concentration is meditation. A number of easy and interesting exercises have been described. The fruit of meditation is Samadhi and this forms the subject-matter of the next lesson. Samadhi is superconscious state, wherein the Yogi gets superintuitional or supersensual knowledge and supersensual bliss. In Samadhi the Yogi communes with the Lord and enjoys Absolute Independence. He has reached the Goal now.

In the Eleventh Lesson I have dealt with the Serpentine Power or the mighty pristine Force underlying all organic and inorganic matter. This Force is in a dormant state and is sleeping a sleep-trance in almost all persons in the basal Muladhara Chakra. When this sleeping Force is roused to action, it pierces through the various centres of spiritual energy in the human body and reaches the crown of the head or the Sahasrara Chakra where She is united with Her Consort, Lord Siva. That Yogi who has taken the sleeping Kundalini to the Sahasrara Chakra and united Her with Lord Siva alone has attained the Goal, not others. The process by which this sleeping Power can be roused to action and taken to the top of the head has also been described with beautiful illustrations. The Yogi who has succeeded in achieving this union becomes the Lord of all powers and knowledge.

In the last Lesson on Spiritual Vibrations and Aura I have stated what vibration and aura mean and various means of producing vibrations of love, joy, peace, mercy, sympathy and purity, and developing the spiritual aura. I have also stated in brief that the human aura has various colours according to the growth and development of a person physically, mentally, morally and spiritually, and that each colour has got its own significance and meaning. The would-be Yogi should dispel all other colours and develop the particular spiritual aura, the colour of which is yellow.

At the end of the book an Appendix has been added and a Glossary of Sanskrit terms given. In appendix 1 a daily routine for aspirants has been chalked out, one for the beginner, another for the intermediate student and a third for the advanced Yogi. I believe that if a similar routine chalked out according to one's own necessity and convenience is followed regularly and systematically, nothing would stand in the way of the aspiring Yogi to achieve success in Yoga. Moreover, he should also maintain a Spiritual Diary similar to the one given in the Appendix realising the importance and benefits of such a discipline. In Appendix II an interesting article on Yoga and Science has also been added in the belief that it would be read with considerable interest.

I appeal to the students of Yoga in the East and the West to start doing some spiritual and Yogic practice in right earnest after digesting and assimilating the truths and ideals inculcated herein, and I hope they would be immensely benefited by this book.

*Sivananda*

# THE UNIVERSAL PRAYER

Thou art, O Lord! the Creator of this universe. Thou art the Protector of this world. Thou art in the grass and the rose. Thou art in the sun and the stars. Salutations unto Thee, O Destroyer of the cycle of births and deaths! Salutations unto Thee, O Bestower of Bliss and Immortality!

O sweet Lord! May I be free from the bonds of Death. May I never again forget my immortal nature. May I be able to look upon all with equal vision. May I attain the Supreme Seat of Brahman. May I be free from impurity and sin. May I know my real essential nature.

Adorations to the Supreme Being who dwells in the hearts of all beings, who is in the fire and water, who is in the plants, herbs and trees, who is in the stones, bricks and iron-bars and who has pervaded the whole universe.

I bow to Thee, O Secret of secrets! I bow to Thee, O Indweller of our hearts! I bow to Thee, O Silent Witness of all activities of all minds! I bow to Thee, O Inner Ruler of all beings! I bow to Thee, O Thread-Soul who connects all beings, who pervades and permeates and interpenetrates all things of this universe!

Salutations to Thee, the Supreme Lord. Thou art without beginning and end. Thou art the flower; Thou art the bee; Thou art woman; Thou art man; Thou art the sea; Thou art the waves; Thou art the old man tottering with a stick; Thou art the saint; and Thou art the rogue.

Thou art Light Divine. Thou art Light of Knowledge. Thou art the Dispeller of darkness. Thou art the Supreme Guru. Thou art beyond the reach of mind and speech. Thou art beyond any kind of limitation. Thou art the Oversoul. Thou art the Self of this universe.

Thou art Self-luminous. Thou art without parts, without actions, without limbs, without any taint of fault, without birth and death. Thou art our Father, Mother, Brother, Friend, Guru, Relative and sole Refuge. Thou art the embodiment of Peace, Bliss, Knowledge, Power, Strength and Beauty.

O All-merciful Lord! Through Thy Grace, may I realise Truth. May I always entertain sublime thoughts. May I realise myself as the Light Divine. May I behold the one sweet immortal Self in all beings. May I realise Brahman with pure understanding.

May that Light of lights ever guide me. May He cleanse my mind of all impurities. May He inspire me. May He bestow on me Power, Courage and Strength. May He remove the veil in the mind. May He remove all obstacles in the Spiritual Path. May He make my life happy and fruitful. I bow to Thee, O Lord of lords, O God of gods, O Deva of devas, O Brahman of the Upanishads, the Support for Maya and Isvara, the Supreme Bridge to Immortality!

*Om Peace! Peace! Peace!*

# INTRODUCTION

The Religion of the Vedanta and Yoga stands forth as a brilliant guiding star to the student of Yoga, Philosophy and Occultism, inviting him to the mysterious unknown world, which he would gladly explore, and encouraging him to march onward until he reaches a stage, when all powers dear to every human heart lie at his command, and all earthly attractions cease to influence him any more. It is a truism that it is in the nature of every human being to strive for happiness, but the happiness he gains by his actions, he finds to his utter dissatisfaction and sorrow, is only of a limited duration. The enjoyments of the senses are transient, and the senses themselves are worn out by excessive enjoyment. Further, sin generally accompanies these enjoyments and makes him unhappy beyond comparison. Even if the pleasures of the world are enjoyed as much as their nature would permit, even if they are as intense, as various, as uninterrupted as possible, yet old age in all its hideous shape threatens him with death and destruction. It should be remembered that the enjoyments of heaven itself are not in reality more enviable than these pleasures of the senses; they are of the same nature though more unmixed and durable. Moreover they also come to an end as they are gained by actions; and as actions are finite, their effect must also be finite. In a word, there is necessarily an end to all these enjoyments.

O little man of little faith! Why do you vainly strive for pleasures, which you know cannot satisfy you beyond the moment of enjoyment? Look out for an unchangeable, infinite and supreme happiness which must come from a Being in whom there is no change. Search and find out such a Being, and if you could only succeed in your quest, then you can get that unaltered happiness from Him.

All the great religions of the world proclaim in one unanimous voice that there is One Being as mentioned above. This Being, believe me, is not very far from you. He is quite close to you. He resides in the body-temple of yours, in the innermost recesses of your heart. He is the silent Witness of your mind, the Watcher of all the activities of your intellect. He is the Supreme Being of the Scriptures so highly eulogised by Saints, Sages, Yogins, Philosophers and Prophets. This Being can be realised by all through the practice of Yoga.

It is a well-known fact that any number of zeros have no intrinsic value unless the No. 1 is placed before them. Even so the wealth of all the three worlds is nothing, if you do not lead a spiritual life, if you do not try to acquire the Spiritual Wealth, if you do not strive for Self-realisation. You will have to live in the Soul or the Self within. You will have to add Atman to the life here. That is the reason why Lord Jesus says: "Seek ye first the Kingdom of God and His righteousness, and all these things shall be added unto you."

Every one of you is a power in yourself. You can influence others. You can radiate Joy and Peace to millions upon millions of people far and near. You can elevate others even from a long distance. You can transmit your powerful, soul-stirring, beneficial thoughts to others, because you are an image of God, nay, you are God

Himself—the moment the veil of ignorance enshrouding you is rent asunder.

This world is a great school. This world is for your education. You learn several valuable lessons daily. If you are wise enough to utilise all opportunities to the best possible advantage in the spirit of Yoga, your capacities and will-power will develop to an astonishing degree. You will grow. You will evolve. You will expand. There will be integral development. You will march forward towards the goal. All veils will drop down one by one. All limitations or barriers will be annihilated. All shackles or fetters will be torn asunder. You will receive more and more Divine Light, Knowledge, Purity, Peace and Spiritual Strength.

You are the author of your own fate. You yourself have created this. You yourself are entirely responsible for this. You are the architect of your joys and sorrows. Just as the spider or the silkworm creates a web or cocoon for its own destruction, so also you have created this cage of flesh by your own actions, attractions, repulsions and false egoism. You have become the slave of the flesh, slave of your body and mind, slave of countless desires. You are sunk in the quagmire of deepest ignorance.

Weep not, my child! Sorrow not! A glorious brilliant future is awaiting you! Strive to come out of this false cage of illusion right now, this very second. If your attempt is true and sincere, if you endeavour with all your might and main to achieve this end, then by the ready Grace of the Lord thou shalt drive away these dark clouds of ignorance and shine in your true divine colours, in your native, pristine glory.

Cast aside the erroneous idea: "I am the body." Develop the consciousness and realisation of the real "I" within you. This real "I" is Sat-Chit-Ananda or Atman or the Self, the one common Consciousness, the spiritual thread that links all hearts.

Awaken yourself to the conscious realisation of your actual oneness with the Supreme Self. Think of the Self continuously. As Tennyson says: "Let thy voice rise like a fountain for me night and day." This is the real spiritual practice (Brahma-abhyasa). This will eventually lead to Self-realisation. Let the struggle be keen. Let your endeavour be sincere. Let your motive be pure. There must be iron discipline, iron determination, iron will and iron Sadhana (spiritual practice). Then there will be no difficulty in the attainment of the final beatitude of life—a life sublime in its nature, resplendent with spiritual light, radiant with splendour, vibrant with ecstasy and replete with Peace.

Mere intellectual conception of this identity or oneness will not serve your purpose. You must actually feel and experience the truth of the same through intuition. You must become fully aware of the Real Self, the basis or substratum or bed-rock of this world, body, mind, Prana and the senses. You must enter into a consciousness in which the realisation becomes part and parcel of your daily life. You must live this ideal spiritual life daily. Let your neighbours actually feel how entirely a changed being you are—a superman. Let them smell the Divine Fragrance from you. A full-blown Yogi can never be concealed. Just as fragrant fumes emanate from scented sticks, so also sweet spiritual fragrance will emanate from your body, the moment you attain perfection in Yoga, even though you may shut yourself up in a cave of the far-off Himalayas.

A Yoga-Bhrashta (one who had fallen from Yogic practices), who did rigorous spiritual Sadhana in his previous birth, but was unable to get Self-realisation on account of some cause or other, gets Self-realisation in this birth like a flash of lightning in the twinkling of an eye. He is a born adept. He does no spiritual practice. He has no spiritual preceptor (Guru). He had his initiation in his previous birth. Ashtavakra and Rishi Vamadeva, the two Yoga-Bhrashtas of yore, attained Knowledge of the Self even while they were in the wombs of their mothers. Jnanadeva of Alandi (a place near Poona, India), author of Jnanesvari-Gita, was a born adept. He exhibited several Siddhis (psychic powers) even when he was a small boy. He touched a buffalo and the buffalo repeated the Vedas. He created fire on his own back and his sister baked bread over it. But such instances are very rare. The vast majority of people should do intense Sadhana before they attain Self-realisation.

The Hindu Sastras assert with astonishing emphasis: "This world of names and forms is unreal; God alone is Real." The objects a man of the world considers precious, a Yogi shuns as worthless. This world with all its variegated pleasures, its pains, its joys, its sorrows, its rivers, mountains, sky, sun, moon, and the stars; with its dukes and beggars exists only in order that the fragments of the one Self embodied in so many forms may regain their lost Divine Consciousness and realise the true pristine glory and manifest the powers of the Self through the matter that envelops them.

There is no such thing as inanimate matter. There is life in every thing. Life is involved in a piece of stone. Matter is vibrant with life. This has been conclusively proved by modern science. Smile with the flowers and the green grass. Play with the butterflies and the cobras. Shake hands with the shrubs, ferns and twigs. Talk to the rainbow, wind, stars and sun. Converse with the running brooks and the turbulent waves of the sea. Keep company with your walking stick and enjoy its sweet company. Develop friendship with all your neighbours, dogs, cats, cows, human beings, trees, in fact, with all nature's creation. Then you will have a wide, perfect, rich, full life. Then you will realise God. Then you will achieve success in Yoga. This state can hardly be described in finite words. It should be felt and experienced by you by unfolding the divinity within.

This remarkable unfolding from the stone to the God goes on through millions of years, through aeons of time. But in the individual this unfolding takes place more rapidly and quickly with all the force of its past behind it. "These forces that manifest and unveil themselves in evolution are cumulative in their power. Embodied in the stone, in the mineral world, they grow and put out a little more strength, and in the mineral world accomplish their unfolding. Then they become too strong for the mineral and press on into the vegetable world. There they unfold more and more of their divinity, until they become too mighty for the vegetable, and become animal. Expanding within and gaining experiences from the animal, they again overflow the limits of the animal and appear as the human. In the human being they still grow and accumulate with ever-increasing force, and exert greater pressure against the barrier; and then out of the human, they press into the superhuman. This last process of evolution is called Yoga." Therefore Yoga, when it is definitely begun, is not something new, as is often imagined.

xix

If you begin to view Yoga in this light, then this Yoga, which looked so foreign and so strange, will appear to wear a familiar face, and come to you in a garb not altogether strange. It will not look so strange that from the man you should pass on to superman, from mortality to immortality, and enter a region where divinity becomes more manifest.

When you begin to learn that there is one Self in all these names and forms, that He is the same in a king or a peasant, in a bird or a beast, in a man or a woman, in a stone or a piece of wood, that all powers seen throughout the world are latent in "inorganic" substances also, that this Self is the same at all times, and that there is no increase or diminution in the Self, then Yoga will become possible of achievement.

In fact you have practised Yoga, consciously or unconsciously, in your previous births, and this is a vital point that should not be lost sight of. All that you have now to do is to give a powerful momentum to quicken the process of unfolding the divinity and attain the Highest Goal of Life—*Perfection, Peace, Joy, Immortality and Happiness.*

In this book I have given definite lines for attaining true success in Yoga. You can also attain happiness, popularity, name, fame, power, wealth, social distinction and all-round smashing success in all your undertakings to an extent that would surprise not only your own self but all others with whom you come in contact. This volume contains the boiled down essence of years of extensive research and personal experience. I assure you that you will be able to fully realise the benefits of Yogic practices by the help of this one book alone. Not a moment should be delayed. You are growing older and older hour by hour.

Three things rare indeed and due to the Grace of God are: a human birth, the longing for Liberation and the protecting care of a perfected Sage. The man who, having by some means, obtained a human birth, with a male body and mastery of the scriptures to boot, is foolish enough not to exert for Self-realisation, verily commits suicide, for he kills himself by clinging to things unreal. Let me sound a note of warning here: You may not get again this rare human birth. Make hay while the sun shines. Go to the Fountain-head of God and drink deep the Nectar of Immortality. May the Lord Krishna, the Lord of the Yogins, the Great Master, shower His choicest blessings upon you all and give you a nice push in the Path of Spirituality is my fervent prayer!

# CONTENTS

# Practical Lessons
## In
## Yoga

# YOGA AND ITS OBJECTS

YOGA Philosophy is one of the six systems of Hindu Philosophy which exist in India. Unlike so many other philosophies of the world, it is a philosophy that is wholly practical. Yoga is an exact science based on certain immutable Laws of Nature. It is well known to people of all countries of the world interested in the study of Eastern civilisation and culture, and is held in awe and reverence as it contains in it the master-key to unlock the realms of Peace, Bliss, Mystery and Miracle. Even the philosophers of the West found solace and peace in this Divine Science. Jesus Christ himself was a Yogi of a superior order, a Raja-Yogi indeed. The founder of the Yoga Philosophy was Patanjali Maharshi, who was not only a Philosopher and a Yogi, but a Physician as well. He is said to have lived about three hundred years before Jesus Christ.

Patanjali defiles Yoga as the suspension of all the functions of the mind. As such, any book on Yoga, which does not deal with these three aspects of the subject, viz., mind, its functions and the method of suspending them, can he safely laid aside as unreliable and incomplete.

The word Yoga comes from the Sanskrit root "Yuj" which means "to join." Yoga is a science that teaches us the method of joining the individual soul and the Supreme

Soul. It is the merging of the individual will with the Cosmic or Universal Will. Yoga is that inhibition of the functions of the mind which leads to the absolute abidance of the soul in its own real nature of Divine Glory and Divine Splendour. It is the process by which the identity of the individual soul and the Oversoul is established by the Yogi. In other words, the human soul is brought into conscious communion with God. Yoga is the Science of sciences, that disentangles the individual soul from the phenomenal world of sense-objects and links with the Absolute, whose inherent attributes are Infinite Bliss, Supreme Peace, Infinite Knowledge and unbroken Joy.

Yoga is that state of Absolute Peace wherein there is neither imagination nor thought. Yoga is control of mind and its modifications. Yoga teaches us how to control the modifications of the mind and attain liberation. It teaches us how to transmute the unregenerate nature and attain the state of Divinity. It is the complete suppression of the tendency of the mind to transform itself into objects, thoughts, etc. Yoga kills all sorts of pain, misery and tribulation. It gives you freedom from the round of births and deaths, with its concomitant evils of disease, old age, etc., and bestows upon you all the Divine Powers and final liberation through super-intuitional knowledge.

The word Yoga is also applicable in its secondary sense to the factors of Yoga, viz., self-training, study, the different actions and practices that go to make up Yoga as they are conducive to the fulfilment of Yoga and as such indirectly lead to emancipation. Union with God is the goal of human life and that ought to become the touchstone of all human endeavours. That is the be-all and end-all of existence.

Equanimity is Yoga. Serenity is Yoga. Skill in actions is Yoga. Control of the senses and the mind is Yoga. Anything by which the best and the highest in life can be attained is also Yoga. Yoga is thus all-embracing, all-inclusive and universal in its application leading to all-round development of body, mind and soul.

The object of Yoga is to weaken what are called the five afflictions. The five afflictions are: Ignorance, Egoism, Likes, Dislikes and the instinct of self-preservation (or clinging to bodily life). Ignorance is the fertile soil which bears an abundant crop of the rest. On account of ignorance only egoism has manifested. Wherever there is egoism, there invariably exist likes, dislikes and the rest side by side. Clinging to bodily life or fear of death is born of likes only. It is nothing but attachment.

Egoism is a specific form of ignorance. The mind gets itself attached wherever there is pleasure. If the mind likes pomegranate, it gets itself attached to this fruit, as it derives pleasure from eating it. The mind runs after things that have been associated with agreeable experiences in the past. This is attachment (like). The mind runs away from objects which have caused pain. This is dislike. These are all the faults of man himself. The world can never hurt you. The five elements are your best teachers. They help you in a variety of ways. The things created by the Lord are all beneficial. It is only the creation of man, that brings pain and misery. These five afflictions bind you to the outside objects and reduce you to piteous slavery. These afflictions remain as tendencies even when they are inoperative. These afflictions and tendencies can be attenuated by Yogic discipline.

On account of ignorance you have forgotten your primitive Divine Glory. On account of this evil you are not able to remember your old status of Godhood, your original immortal, blissful, divine nature. Ignorance is the root cause of egoism, likes, dislikes and the rest. These five afflictions are great impediments to Yoga. They stand as stumbling-blocks to the attainment of Self-realisation.

These five afflictions remain in a dormant, attenuated, overpowered or fully developed state. When the husband begins to quarrel with the wife, his love for her becomes dormant and he shows dislike for her for the time being. In a Yogic student these afflictions become thinned out or attenuated by the spiritual force of his Yogic practices. But they do exist in a subtle state. They cannot do any havoc. They are like the cobra whose poisonous fangs have been extracted by the snake-charmer. The "overpowered state" is that state in which one set of impressions is kept under restraint for some time by another powerful set of impressions; but they manifest again, when the cause of the suppression is removed. In a worldly man with passions and appetites these can be seen operating in fullest swing. But in a fully developed or full-blown Yogi these afflictions and impressions are burnt in toto.

Owing to ignorance you have mistaken the physical body for the Self and this is all the mistake you have committed. But it is a serious mistake indeed. By changing your mental outlook, by purifying your heart and intellect, you can attain Knowledge of Self. Mind, Prana, body and the senses are all instruments only. The real Seer is the Self who is pure, unchanging, eternal, self-luminous, self-existent, self-contained, infinite and immortal. When you begin to identify yourself with this immortal, all-pervading Self, all miseries will come to an end.

Likes and dislikes are the causes for doing good and evil deeds. Good and evil deeds bring pleasure and pain. Thus the round of births and deaths is kept from time immemorial by the six-spoked wheel of Likes, Dislikes, Virtue, Vice, Pleasure and Pain.

The Yogic student should first try to weaken these five afflictions. Three practices are prescribed for this purpose. They are: Austerity (Tapas), Study of Scriptures (Svadhyaya) and Resignation to the Will of the Lord (Isvara-pranidhana). The practitioner should have intense faith in the efficacy of his practices. Then the energy to carry on with the practices will manifest by itself. Then the real memory will dawn. When there is memory, then there is no difficulty in practising concentration. If there is concentration, discrimination will dawn. That is the reason why Patanjali says: "Samadhi will come through faith, energy, memory, concentration and discrimination."

Therefore, to get success in concentration, meditation and the practice of Yoga, you must have tremendous patience, tremendous will and tremendous perseverance. Plunge yourself in concentration. Merge the mind in the one idea of God and God alone. Let the mind fully get absorbed there. Forget other things. Let the whole body, muscles, tissues, nerves, cells and brain be filled with the one idea of

God. This is the way to positive success. Great sages and saints of yore have practised Yoga in this way only. Work hard. You will reach the goal. You will also become a great saint. Whatever one has achieved can be achieved by others also. This is the Law.

## LESSON II

# YOGA SADHANA

SADHANA means any spiritual practice that aids the aspirant to realise God. It is a means to attain the goal of life. Without Sadhana no one can achieve the goal. Sadhana differs according to taste, temperament and capacity.

You can realise the goal of life by four different paths. Just as one and the same coat will not suit Mr. John, Mr. Smith, Mr. Dick and Mr. Williams, so also one path will not suit all people. These four paths lead to the same goal, viz., the attainment of the Ultimate Reality. Roads are different but the destination is the same. Lord Krishna says to Arjuna: "Howsoever men approach Me, even so do I reward them, for, the path men take from every side, is Mine, O Partha." The four paths are: the path of work (Karma-Yoga), the path of devotion or love (Bhakti-Yoga), the path of psychic control (Raja-Yoga) and the path of self-analysis and knowledge (Jnana-Yoga).

These divisions are not hard and fast. There is no line of demarcation between one another. One path does not exclude the other. For instance Karma-Yoga is suitable for a man of active temperament; Bhakti-Yoga for a man of emotional temperament; Raja-Yoga for a man of mystic temperament; and the path of Jnana-Yoga or Vedanta for a man of will or reason. Each path blends into the other.

Ultimately they all converge and become one. Thus it is hard to say where Raja-Yoga ends and Jnana-Yoga begins. All aspirants of different paths meet on a common platform in the long run.

Religion must educate and develop the whole man—his head, heart and hand. Then only there will be perfection. One-sided development is not commendable. The four paths, far from being antagonistic to one another, indicate that the different methods of the Yoga System are in absolute harmony with each other. Karma-Yoga leads to Bhakti-Yoga which in its turn leads to Raja-Yoga. Raja-Yoga brings Jnana. Supreme devotion is Jnana only. Bhakti, it should be borne in mind, is not divorced from Jnana. On the contrary, Jnana intensifies Bhakti. Karma-Yoga removes the tossing of mind, Raja-Yoga steadies the mind and Jnana-Yoga removes the veil of ignorance and brings in the Knowledge of Self. Every Yoga is a fulfilment of the preceding one. Thus Bhakti is the fulfilment of Karma, Yoga of Bhakti, and Jnana of all the preceding three.

The practice of Karma-Yoga prepares the aspirant for the reception of Knowledge of Self. It moulds him into a proper Adhikari (aspirant) for the study of Vedanta. Ignorant people jump at once to Jnana-Yoga without having any preliminary training in Karma-Yoga. That is the reason why they fail miserably to realise Truth. The impurities still lurk in their minds. The mind is filled with likes and dislikes. They only *talk* of Brahman or God. They indulge in all sorts of useless discussions, vain debates and dry, endless controversies. Their philosophy is on their lips only.

In other words, they are lip-Vedantins. What is really wanted is *practical* Vedanta through ceaseless selfless service.

Those who follow the path of Karma-Yoga should do work for work's sake, without any motive. Two things are indispensable requisite in the practice of Karma-Yoga. A Karma-Yogi should have extreme non-attachment for the fruits of his works and secondly he should dedicate all his actions at the Altar of God with the feeling of Isvararpana (self-surrender). Non-attachment brings freedom and immortality. Attachment is death. Non-attachment is eternal life. Non-attachment makes a man absolutely fearless. When you thus consecrate all your actions to the Lord, you will naturally develop devotion towards Him, and the greater the devotion the nearer you are to the Lord. You will slowly begin to feel that God directly works through your body and senses. You will feel no strain in the discharge of your works now. The heavy load you felt previously on account of your false egoism, has now vanished out of sight, never to return.

The doctrine of Karma-Yoga[1] forms an integral part of Vedanta. It expounds the riddle of life and the riddle of the universe. It brings solace, satisfaction and happiness to one and all. It is a self-evident truth. Fortunately even the Westerners have begun to acknowledge its importance and veracity. They have no other go. Every sensible man or woman will have to accept it. "As you sow, so you reap"

---

1   For detailed particulars vide my book *Practice of Karma-Yoga.*

holds good not only on the physical plane but in the moral world as well. Every thought and every deed of yours generate in you certain tendencies which will affect your life herein and hereafter. If you do good actions in a selfless spirit, you will naturally soar high to regions of bliss and peace. Karma-Yoga is the lowest rung in the Spiritual Ladder; but it lifts us up to ineffable heights. It destroys pride, selfishness and egoism. It helps growth and evolution.

Every work is a mixture of good and evil. This world of ours is a relative plane. You must therefore strive to do such actions that can bring maximum of good and minimum of evil. If you know the secret of work, the technique of Karma-Yoga, you will be absolutely free from the taint of Karma. That secret is to work without attachment and egoism. The central teaching of the Bhagavad-Gita and the Yoga-Vasishtha is non-attachment to work. Lord Krishna says to Arjuna: "O Arjuna, work incessantly. Your duty is to work always. But do not expect fruits. The lot of that man who expects fruits is pitiable. He is the most miserable man in the world."

Generally people have various motives when they work. Some work in society for getting name and fame, some for money, some for getting power and position, and some others for getting enjoyments in heaven. Some build temples and churches with the idea that their sins will be washed off. Some perform sacrifices for getting children. Some sink wells and tanks so that their names will be remembered even after their death. Some lay out gardens and public parks with the idea that they will enjoy such lovely parks and gardens in heaven. Some do acts of charity with the idea that they will be born in the house of a Henry Ford or a Rockefeller in their next birth.

The greatest service that one can render to another is the imparting of Knowledge of Self. Spiritual help is the highest of all. The root cause for all suffering is ignorance (Avidya) only. Cut the knot of Avidya and drink the sweet Nirvanic Bliss. That sage who tries to remove the ignorance of men is the greatest benefactor in the world. If you remove the hunger of man, it is after all a temporary physical help. It is removal of physical want for three or four hours. Then again the hunger manifests. The man remains in the same miserable state. Thus it is safe to conclude that building of hospitals, poor-houses, *dharmasalas* or choultries for distribution of free food, clothes, etc., is not the highest kind of help, though they are absolutely necessary. I say this is not the highest kind of help, because I ask: How long can these last? Miseries have to be eradicated once and forever. The world will remain in the same miserable state even if you build millions of hospitals and feeding-places. There is something that can put an end to all these miseries, sufferings, worries and anxieties, and that something is Knowledge of Self.

Bhakti-Yoga[2] is the path of devotion or the path of affection that is suitable for people of devotional temperament or in whom the love-element predominates. Ladies are fit for this path, for affection predominates in

2   For detailed particulars vide my book *Practice of Bhakti-Yoga.*

them. Generally there is an admixture of devotional and intellectual temperaments in all persons. Hence Bhakti-Yoga is suitable for the vast majority of persons. In Bhakti-Yoga the devotee makes absolute and unreserved self-surrender. He depends upon the Lord for everything. He is extremely humble and meek. He develops devotion to the Lord gradually to a very high degree by repeating the Name of the Lord, studying the Holy Scriptures and practising the nine modes of devotion. Hearing the Name of the Lord, singing His praises, remembering His presence, serving His Lotus-Feet, worshipping Him, bowing before Him, attending on Him, loving Him as a Friend and surrendering of the self entirely to Him are the nine modes of devotion. The devotee will observe austerities, pray frequently to Him and offer mental worship to Him. He will serve his fellow-men realising that the Lord dwells in the hearts of all. This is the Sadhana for those who wish to tread the path of Yoga of devotion.

Sri Sankara, the great Advaita Jnani, was a great Bhakta of Lord Hari, Hara and Devi. Jnanadeva of Alandi, a great Yogi of late, was a Bhakta of Lord Krishna. Ramakrishna Paramahamsa worshipped Kali and got Jnana through Swami Totapuri, his Advaita Guru. Appayya Dikshitacharya, a famous Jnani of South India, author of "Siddhanta Lesha" and other monumental works on Vedanta, was a devotee of Lord Siva.

It behoves, therefore, that Bhakti can be combined with much advantage with Jnana. Bhakti is a means to an end. It gives purity of mind and removes mental oscillation (Vikshepa). Sakama Bhakti (devotion with expectation) brings Svarga for the devotee, while Nishkama Bhakti (devotion without expectation) brings purity of mind and Jnana.

A life without love of God is practical death. There is no power greater than love. You can win the hearts of others through love alone. You can conquer your enemies through love alone. You can tame wild animals through love alone. The glory of love is ineffable. Its splendour is indescribable. The power of love is unfathomable.

True religion does not consist in ritualistic observances, baths and pilgrimages but in loving all. Cosmic Love is all-embracing and all-inclusive. In the presence of pure love all distinctions and differences, all hatred, jealousy and egoism are dispelled just as darkness is dispelled by the penetrating rays of the morning sun. There is no religion higher than Love. There is no knowledge higher than Love. There is no treasure higher than Love, because Love is Truth, Love is God. This world came out of Love; it exists in Love and it will ultimately dissolve in Love. A heart without love is a desert without water. God is an ocean of Love. In every corner of His creation, you can see ample evidence of His unbounded Love for His children.

It is all so easy to talk of Universal Love, but when you come to the practical field, you manifestly show signs of failure. If Mr. John speaks ill of you and uses harsh words, you are thrown out of balance instantaneously. You get irritated, show your angry face and pay him in the same coin. You do not like to part with your possessions, when you see people in distress. A man who is struggling to develop Cosmic Love and realise Him through Love cannot keep anything for himself more than he actually needs for keeping his life going peacefully. He will willingly sacrifice even this little to serve a needy person and undergo starvation with much pleasure. He will rejoice that the Lord has given him a wonderful opportunity to serve Him. People generally *talk* of Universal Love but are very niggardly in *action*. They show lip-sympathy and lip-love in mere words. This is nothing short of hypocrisy.

Those who talk of Universal Love should endeavour to develop various good qualities. They should serve humanity untiringly day and night with disinterested, selfless spirit for many years. They must be prepared to bear calmly insults and injuries. Then only there is a prospect of developing Cosmic Love. Otherwise it is all vain, flowery talk and idle-gossiping only.

The saints, seers and prophets of the world have spoken of Love as the end and aim of life. Lord Krishna has preached Love through His flute. Lord Buddha was an ocean of Love. He gave up His body to appease the hunger of a tiger's cub. Raja Sibi gave flesh equal to the weight of a pigeon from his own breast to satisfy the appetite of a hawk. Lord Rama lived a life of Love and showed Love in every inch of His activity. Lord Jesus also preached and practised Love in the fullest measure.

O dear children of Love! Draw inspiration from their teachings and tread the path of Love. Remember Him. Feel His indwelling presence everywhere. See Him in all faces, in all objects, in all movements, in all feelings, in all sentiments, in all actions. Meditate upon His form with single-minded devotion. Become a peerless devotee of the Lord in this very life, nay in this very second.

The student treading the path of Raja-Yoga[3] has to ascend the Spiritual Ladder step by step, stage by stage. There are eight limbs in Raja-Yoga, viz., Yama, Niyama, Asana, Pranayama, Pratyahara, Dharana, Dhyana and Samadhi. By practising Yama and Niyama at the outset the student gets ethical training and purification of mind. By developing friendship, mercy and complacency, he destroys hatred, jealousy and harshness of heart and thereby gets peace of mind. By practising Asana he steadies his posture and gets complete control and mastery over his body. Then he practises Pranayama to remove the tossing of mind and destroy Rajas (passion) and Tamas (inertia). His body becomes light and elastic. By practising Pratyahara (withdrawal of the Indriyas or senses from sensual objects) he gets strength and peace of mind. Now he is fit for concentration which comes of itself. He practises meditation and enters into Samadhi. By the combined practice of concentration, meditation and Samadhi (Yogic Samyama), he gets various Siddhis (powers). By concentration on the senses, egoism, mind, etc., he gets various other powers and experiences. He now sees without eyes, tastes without tongue, hears without ears, smells without a nose and feels without a skin. He can work miracles. He simply wills and everything comes into being.

3 For detailed particulars vide my book *Raja-Yoga.*

Those who follow the path of Jnana-Yoga or Vedanta[4] should first acquire the four means of salvation, viz., Viveka, Vairagya, Shat-Sampatti and Mumukshutva. Viveka is discrimination between the Real and the unreal. Vairagya is indifference or dispassion for sensual objects herein and hereafter. Shat-Sampatti is the sixfold virtue, viz., Sama, (calmness of mind), Dama (restraint of the senses), Uparati (satiety), Titiksha (power of endurance), Sraddha (faith) and Samadhana (one-pointedness of mind). Mumukshutva is intense longing for liberation. Then they should approach· a Brahma-Nishtha Guru (one who is established in Brahman or God), who has fully realised the Supreme Self and hear the Scriptures directly from his mouth. Then they should reflect and meditate on what they heard and attain Self-realisation. Now the Jnani exclaims in exuberant joy: "The Atman alone is, One without a second. Atman or the Self is the one Reality. I am Brahman (Aham Brahma Asmi). I am Siva (Sivoham). I am He (Sivoham)." He, the liberated soul, sees the Self in all beings and all beings in the Self.

There are also three other forms of Yoga in addition to the four mentioned above. These are: Hatha-Yoga, Mantra-Yoga and Laya-Yoga or Kundalini-Yoga. Hatha-Yoga relates to the physical body, Asanas, Bandhas, Mudras, Pranayama, vow of silence, steady-gazing, crystal-gazing, standing on one leg, etc. Hatha-Yoga is not separate from Raja-Yoga. It prepares the student to take up Raja-Yoga. Hatha-Yoga and Raja-Yoga are, therefore, the

---

4   For detailed particulars vide my book Vedanta in Daily Life.

necessary counterparts of each other. No one can become a Yogi of a perfect order without a clear knowledge of the practice of the two Yogas. Raja-Yoga begins where properly practised Hatha-Yoga ends. A Hatha-Yogi starts his Sadhana with his body and Prana (breath); a Raja-Yogi with his mind. A Hatha-Yogi gets different powers when the mighty Kundalini-Sakti reaches the Sahasrara Chakra (at the top of the head); a Raja-Yogi gets psychic powers by the combined practice of concentration, meditation and Samadhi at one and the same time. Mantra-Yoga relates to the recitation of certain Mantras (sacred words to which definite powers are ascribed), such as *Om Namo Narayanaya, Om Namo Bhagavate Vasudevaya* and *Om Namah Sivaya.* Laya-Yoga is Kundalini-Yoga. Concentration on the sound emanating from the heart-lotus is Laya-Yoga. Laya is dissolution. The mind is dissolved in God just as a lump of ice is dissolved in a tumbler of soda-water.

A Jnana-Yogi can practise his Sadhana even while walking, eating and talking. He is not in need of any Asana or room. But a Raja-Yogi wants a room and an Asana for his practice. A Jnana-Yogi is always in Samadhi. He is not affected by Maya or illusion. There is no 'in Samadhi' and 'out of Samadhi' for a Jnani, whereas a Yogi is affected by Maya when he comes down from his Samadhi. A Raja-Yogi plugs his mind, as it were, through effort, just as you plug a bottle with a cork, and thus stops all mental activities. He tries to make the mind quite blank. He remains as a silent witness of all the activities of his mind and intellect. A Raja-Yogi commences his practice with his mind. A Jnana-Yogi starts his practices with his will and reason.

A Karma-Yogi does selfless service to kill his little self. A Bhakta or devotee of the Lord practises self-surrender to annihilate his egoism. A .Jnani practises self-denial. The methods are different but all want to destroy this self-arrogating little "I", the root cause of bondage and suffering. Karma-Yoga prepares the mind for the reception of Light and Knowledge. It expands the heart *ad infinitum*. It breaks all barriers that stand in the way of unity and oneness. Bhakti and meditation are also mental Karmas. There can be no Jnana without Yoga. The fruit of Bhakti is Jnana. Have you now understood the nature of the four Yogas and their interrelations?

There is a verse in Sanskrit the gist of which runs as follows: "The Sastras are endless; there is much to be known; time is short; obstacles are many; that which is the essence should be grasped just as the swan does in the case of milk mixed with water." I therefore want you to start doing some kind of spiritual practice or other and realise the goal of life and justify your existence before the Lord on the "Day of Judgment."[5]

---

5 See Lesson XI

# YOGIC DISCIPLINE[6]

YOGA is rooted in virtue. Ethical discipline is very necessary for success in Yoga. Ethical discipline is the practice of right conduct in life. The two moral back-bones of Yoga are Yama and Niyama, which the aspirant must practise in his daily life. These correspond roughly to the ten commandments of Lord Jesus or to the noble eightfold path of Lord Buddha. Non-injuring (Ahimsa), truthfulness (Satyam), non-stealing (Asteya), continence (Brahmacharya) and non-covetousness (Aparigraha) are the component parts of Yama. Internal and external purification (Saucha), contentment (Santosha), austerity (Tapas), study of religious and philosophical books (Svadhyaya) and self-surrender to the Lord (Isvara-Pranidhana) come under Niyama. Practice of Yama and Niyama will eradicate all the impurities of the mind. In fact, Yama and Niyama form the corner-stones of Yoga philosophy.

Pre-eminence is given to abstention from injuring any living creature (Ahimsa) amongst all other virtues. There must be non-injuring in thought, word and deed.

---

6  A lecture delivered in the Hallett Hall, Gaya, by Swami Sivananda Sarasvati on March 3, 1937.

Non-injuring is placed first because it is the source of the following nine. The practice of universal love or brotherhood is nothing but the practice of non-injuring. He who practises non-injuring will get quick success in Yoga. The practitioner must abandon even harsh words and unkind looks. He must show goodwill and friendliness to one and all. He must respect life. He must remember that one common Self dwells in the hearts of all beings.

Truthfulness (Satyam) comes next in order. Thought must agree with word, and word with action. This is truthfulness. These virtues are attainable only by the unselfish. Truth can hardly arise unless there is pure motive behind all actions. The word of the Yogi must be a blessing to others.

Then comes non-stealing (Asteya). You must be satisfied with what you get by honest means. The Law of Karma is inexorable. You will have to suffer for every wrong action of yours. Action and reaction are equal and opposite. Amassing wealth is really theft. The whole wealth of all the three worlds belongs to the Lord. You are only a caretaker of his wealth. You must willingly share what you have with all and spend it in charity.

The fourth virtue is the practice of celibacy. That portion of human energy which is expressed in sexual union when controlled, becomes transmuted into a form of special spiritual energy called Ojas-Sakti and this is stored up in the brain. If you practise Yoga and at the same time lead an impure, voluptuous and immoderate life, how can you expect progress in Yoga? All great spiritual giants of the world have practised celibacy and that is the reason why they were able to thrill and electrify the whole world through the power of the special spiritual energy they had stored up in their brains. A Yogi with an abundance of this energy keeps his audience spell-bound, as it were, and sways them even as a monarch sways his dominions. There is a peculiar charm in his smile and power in the words emanating from his heart. He produces a very profound impression in the minds of all with whom he comes in contact.

Householders are allowed to visit their wives once in a month at the proper time, without the idea of sexual enjoyment, but just for the sake of preservation of progeny. If this rule is observed, then it tantamounts to the practice of celibacy. Such observers of this rule are also Brahmacharins. As soon as a son is born, the wife becomes the mother, because the father himself is born in the form of the son. A son is nothing but the modified energy of the father.

Brahmacharya is the basis of acquiring immortality. Brahmacharya brings material progress and psychic advancement. Brahmacharya is the substratum for a life in the Atman. It is a potent weapon for waging a relentless war against the internal monsters—passion, greed, anger, miserliness, hypocrisy, etc. It contributes to perennial joy and uninterrupted, undecaying bliss. It gives tremendous energy, clear brain, gigantic will-power, bold understanding, retentive memory and good power of enquiry (Vichara-Sakti). It is through Brahmacharya and Brahmacharya alone that you can have physical, mental, moral and spiritual advancement.

What is wanted is restraint and not suppression of sexual desire. In restraint no sexual thought will arise in the mind. There is perfect sublimation of sex-energy. But in suppression the aspirant is not safe. There *are* sexual thoughts. When favourable opportunities occur, the repressed desire manifests with redoubled force and vengeance, and there is the danger of a miserable downfall. One should be very careful.

After Dhanvantari had taught all the secrets of the Ayurveda system of medicine to his disciples, they enquired the key-note of this science. The master replied: "I tell you that Brahmacharya is truly a precious jewel; it is the one most effective medicine, nectar indeed, which destroys disease, decay and death. For attaining peace, brightness, memory, knowledge, health and Self-realisation, one should observe Brahmacharya which is the highest duty. Brahmacharya is the highest knowledge; Brahmacharya is the greatest strength. Of the nature of Brahmacharya is verily this Atman, and in Brahmacharya It resides. Saluting Brahmacharya first, the cases beyond cure I cure. Aye, Brahmacharya can undo all the inauspicious signs."

What is wanted is deep inner life. Silence the bubbling thoughts. Keep the mind cool and calm. Open yourself to higher spiritual consciousness. Feel the Divine Presence and Divine Guidance. Fix your mind at the Lotus-Feet of the Lord. Become like a child. Speak to Him freely. Become absolutely candid. Do not hide your thoughts. You cannot do so, because He is the Inner Ruler (Antaryamin). He watches all your thoughts. Pray for Mercy, Light,

Purity, Strength, Peace and Knowledge. You will surely get them. You will be established in Brahmacharya.

A Yogic student should abstain from greed. He should not receive luxurious presents from anybody. Gifts affect the mind of the receiver. These five virtues must be practised in thought, word and deed, for they are not merely restraints but change the character of the practitioner, implying inward purity and strength.

Besides these, the would-be Yogi should also practise certain other active virtues such as cleanliness of body and mind, contentment, austerity, study of religious and philosophical books and self-surrender to God. Contentment does not mean satisfaction, but willingness to accept things as they are and to make the best of them. Austerities like occasional fasting and observance of silence increase the power of endurance. Self-surrender is the regarding of every work as that of the Supreme Lord and renouncing all claims to its fruits. Study of religious books fills the mind with piety and purity. Such a rigorous ethical discipline brings a sense of freedom and moral elevation. When you are sufficiently advanced in the above practices, you can face every temptation by calling in the aid of pure and restraining thoughts.

Two things are necessary for attaining success in mind-control, viz., practice (Abhyasa) and dispassion (Vairagya).

You must try your extremest level best to be free from any desire for any pleasure, seen or unseen, and this dispassion can be attained through constant perception of evil in them. Dispassion is renunciation of attainment. It is aversion to sensual enjoyments herein and hereafter. The dispassion or detachment is of two kinds, the lower and the higher. Vijnana Bhikshu distinguishes the superior and the inferior types of Vairagya in the following way: "The former is a distaste for the good things of life, here or hereafter, due to the experience that they cannot be acquired or preserved without trouble while their loss causes pain and that the quest is never free from egoistic feelings. The latter, however, is based on a clear perception of the difference between intelligence and the objects that appear in its light."

There are various stages in dispassion. The determination to refrain from enjoying all sorts of sensual objects is the first stage. In the second stage certain objects lose their charm for the spiritual aspirant and he attempts to destroy the attraction for others also. In the third stage the senses are controlled, but a vague longing for the sensual enjoyment remains in the mind. In the fourth the aspirant loses completely all interest whatsoever in the external objects. The final stage is a state of highest desirelessness. It is this kind of dispassion that bestows Absolute Independence on the Yogi. In this stage the Yogi renounces all kinds of psychic powers even such as Omniscience, etc.

It is by practice and dispassion that the passage of thought towards external objects can be checked. Mere indifference will not serve the purpose. Practice is also necessary. Remembering God always is also practice. Lord Krishna says to Arjuna with reference to this practice of controlling the mind: "Abandoning without reserve all desires born of the imagination by the mind, curbing in the aggregate of the senses on every side, little by little let him gain tranquillity by means of Reason controlled by steadiness; having made the mind abide in the Self, let him not think of anything. As often as the wavering and unsteady mind goeth forth, so often reining it in, let him bring it under control of the Self." (Bhagavad-Gita: VI-21, 25, 26).

Sound and other objects make the mind wander away. Mind is drawn towards external objects by the force of desire. By convincing oneself of the illusoriness of sense-objects through an investigation into their nature and by cultivating indifference to worldly objects, the mind can be restrained and brought back to the Self to abide finally. In virtue of this practice of Yoga, the Yogi's mind attains peace in the Self. Practice consists in constantly repeating the same idea or thought regarding any object. By constant reflection and exercise of will-power, suggestions should be given to the sub-conscious mind not to look for enjoyment in the changing world without, but in the changeless within. You should exercise great vigilance to get hold of opportunities, when the mind dwells on sense-objects, and suggests to it new meanings and interpretations and make it change its attitude towards them with a view to its ultimate· withdrawal therefrom. This is called practice.

The chief characteristic of the mind in the waking state is to have some object before it to dwell upon. It can never remain blank. It can concentrate on one object at a time. It constantly changes its objects and so it is restless. It· is impetuous, strong and difficult to bend. It is as hard to curb it as the wind. That is the reason why Patanjali Maharshi says that the practice must be steady and continuous and it must stretch over a considerable period and be undertaken with a perfect faith in its regenerating and uplifting powers. You must not show any slackening symptoms at any stage of practice.

Restraint does not come in a day, but by long and continued practice with zeal and enthusiasm. The progress in Yoga can only be gradual. Many people give up the practice of concentration after some time, when they do not see any tangible prospect of getting psychic powers. They become impatient. They do little and expect much. This is bad. Doing any kind of practice by fits and starts will not bring the desired fruit. Direct experience is the goal of life. Though the effort or practice is painful in the beginning, yet it brings Supreme Joy in the end. Lord Krishna says to Arjuna: "Supreme joy is for this Yogi, whose mind is peaceful, whose passionate nature is controlled, who is sinless, and of the nature of the eternal." (Bhagavad-Gita: Ch. VI-27).

Control your senses. Calm your mind. Still the bubbling thoughts. Fix the mind in the lotus of the heart. Concentrate. Meditate. Realise Him intuitively this very second and enjoy the Bliss of the Self.

Have firm and unshakable faith in the existence of God, the supreme, undying, intelligent Principle or Essence or Substance who exists in the three periods of time—past, present and future. He has neither beginning, middle nor end. He is Sat-Chit-Ananda (Existence Absolute, Knowledge Absolute and Bliss Absolute).

O ignorant man! Why do you vainly search for happiness in the perishable external objects of the world conditioned in time, space and causation? You have no peace of mind. Your desires are never fully gratified. You may amass boundless wealth, beget beautiful babies, earn titles, honours, name, fame, power, publicity and all you want, and yet your mind is restless. You have no real, abiding happiness. You feel you still want something. You have no feeling of fullness. Never, therefore, forget from this moment onwards that this feeling of fullness or eternal satisfaction can be obtained only in God by realising Him through constant practice of self-control, purity, concentration, meditation and practice of Yoga.

There is restlessness everywhere. Selfishness, greed, jealousy and lust are playing unimaginable havoc in every heart. Fights, skirmishes and petty quarrels are polluting the atmosphere of the world and creating discord, disharmony and unrest. The bugle is blown and the armies march to the battlefield to destroy their enemies. One nation wages war against another nation for acquiring more dominions and power. Side by side with these bloody wars, peace movement is also working for bringing harmony and peace, for eradicating dire ignorance, the root cause of all human sufferings and for disseminating Divine Knowledge.

The greatest need of the world today is the message of love. Kindle the light of love in your own heart first. Love all. Include all creatures in the warm embrace of your love. Nations can be united by pure love only. World-wars can be put an end to by pure love only. The League of Nations cannot do much. Love is a mysterious divine glue that

unites the hearts of all. It is a magical healing balm of very
high potency. Charge every action with pure love. Kill
cunningness, greed, crookedness and selfishness. It is
extremely cruel to take away the lives of others by using
poisonous gas. This is a capital crime. The scientist who
manufactures the gas in the laboratory cannot escape
without being punished for this crime by the great Lord.
Forget not the Day of Judgement. What will you say unto
the Lord, O ye mortals, who run after power, dominions
and wealth? Have a clean conscience and pure love. You
will verily enter into the Kingdom of God.

How mysterious is the universe! How mysterious are
the silent workings of the unseen Power, who prompts
passionate people to wage wars on the one side and pious
people to disseminate Divine Knowledge on the other and
bring peace and happiness to the suffering humanity at
large!

Desire is the real enemy of peace. Restlessness is fed
by desire just as fire is fed by oil. In the Yoga-Vasishtha
you will find Sage Vasishtha saying to his royal disciple
Rama: "O best of intellects! the obliteration of latent desire,
Gnosis and the dissolution of the mind, if attempted
simultaneously for a sufficient length of time, bestow the
desired fruit." Lord Krishna also says to his royal disciple
Arjuna on the battlefield of Kurukshetra: "It is desire, it is
wrath, begotten by the quality of mobility; all-consuming,
all-polluting, know thou this as our foe here on earth. As a
flame is enveloped by smoke, as a mirror by dust, as an
embryo by the amnion, so is wisdom enveloped by it.
Enveloped is wisdom by this constant enemy the wise in the

form of desire which is insatiable as a flame. Mastering first the senses, slay thou, O mighty armed, the enemy in the form of desire, destructive of wisdom and knowledge."

Swami Vidyaranya Sarasvati, the reputed author of "Panchadasi" and "Jivanmukti-Viveka" says: "So long as these three (obliteration of latent desire, Gnosis and the dissolution of the mind) are not well attempted repeatedly, the state of Jivanmukti (liberation in this life) cannot be realised, even after the lapse of hundreds of years." When the mind is dissolved and there is no sensation of any external cause which can fully rouse mental impressions, latent desire fades away. When latent desire fades away, and there remains no cause for that functioning of the mind which we call lust, anger, etc., the mind is also dissolved. When the mind is annihilated, Gnosis will arise.

The Hindu Scriptures maintain: "Mind alone is, to man, the cause of bondage or liberation; lost in enjoyment, it leads to bondage; freed from the objective, it leads to liberation. As mind freed from the objective leads to liberation, one desirous of liberation or success in the path of Yoga must always try to wipe off the objective from the plane of his mind. When the mind severed from all connections with sensual objects and confined to the light of the heart, finds itself in Ecstasy, it is said to have reached its culminating point. The mind should be prevented from functioning, till its dissolution is attained in the heart; this is Gnosis; this is concentration; the rest is all mere logomachy."

Desire may be described as the hankering for things, which gains such mastery over the mind as to preclude even enquiring into their antecedents and consequences. Man at once becomes that which he identifies himself with, by force of strong and deep attachment and loses memory of everything else in the act. The man, thus subdued by desire, fixing his eye on everything and anything, is deluded into believing it as the real thing. Due to loss of control man perceives everything with beclouded eyes in this deluded fashion, like one under the influence of a strong intoxicant.

As you think, so you become. Think you are a High Court judge, High Court judge you will become. Think you are the monarch of the whole world, monarch of the whole world you will become. Think you are a great teacher, teacher you will become. Think you are poor and weak, poor and weak you will become. Think you are a multi-millionaire, multi-millionaire you will become. Think you are a Yogi, Yogi you will become. Think you are a saint of spotless character, saint of spotless character you will become. Think you are God or Atman or Brahman, God or Atman or Brahman you will become. The whole universe is governed by this wonderful Law of Nature.

Always think rightly and act rightly. Never try to seize the possessions of others. Never envy your neighbours. Entertain noble and sublime thoughts. Have supreme self-confidence and courage. Whatever you do, do it with a will to succeed. You will, by all means, succeed in all your endeavours. Success is yours. You will know of no failures. This is the Sovereign secret. Meditate upon this Secret daily in the morning for some time and enjoy the Bliss of the Self.

In the Vishnupurana you will find: "If the deluded fool loves the body, a mere collection of flesh, blood, pus, faeces, urine, muscles, fat and bones, he will verily love hell itself! To him who is not disgusted with the nasty smell from his own body, what other argument need be adduced for detachment?"

It is a well-known fact that enjoyment cannot bring you satisfaction of desire. On the contrary, it aggravates desire and makes man more restless. The root-cause of all human sufferings and miseries is the craving for worldly enjoyments. The more you hanker after these sensual enjoyments, the more unhappy do you become. The desires also grow when they are not fulfilled. You can never be happy as long as the craving for enjoyments exists.

Desire is born of ignorance (Avidya). Attachment, longing and preference are the constituents of desire. Do not endeavour to fulfil desires. Try to reduce your desires, as best as you can. Withdraw the fuel of gratification. Then the fire of desire will get extinguished by itself. Just as a gheeless lamp dies out, when the ghee is withdrawn, even so the fire of desire will die when the fuel of gratification is withdrawn. If attachment is eradicated, then longing and preference for objects will die by themselves.

Man commits various kinds of sins and injures others when he exerts to get the desired objects. He has to reap the fruits of his actions; hence he is brought again and again in this round of births and deaths. If you increase one object in the list of your possessions or wants, the desire also increases ten times. The more worldly objects you possess, the more distant you are from God. Your mind will always be thinking and planning as to how to get and guard the objects, how to earn tons of money and keep them safe. If the acquired objects are lost, your mind is completely upset. Cares, worries, anxieties and all sorts of mental torments increase with the objects. No doubt, it is painful to earn money. It is more painful to keep the money that is earned. It is still more painful, if the money gets reduced. And it is extremely painful, if the whole money is lost. Money is the abode of all sorts of pain. That is the reason why in India a Sadhu or a Sannyasin does not possess anything. In his grand vision, he does not possess his body also. He constantly asserts. "The body is not mine; I am not body." A real Sannyasin is one who feels: "I am bodiless." These Sannyasins lead a life of perfect dispassion and ruthless renunciation. Renunciation brings in its train supreme Peace.

It is very difficult to become absolutely desireless. A liberated sage or a full-blown Yogi alone is entirely free from the taint of desires, for he has completely annihilated his mind and is enjoying the supreme Bliss of the Self within. How can desires arise in him who is plunged in the ocean of Divine Bliss?

A neophyte in the spiritual path should entertain noble desires. He should do virtuous actions. He should develop intense longing for liberation. In order to achieve this end, he should study the Holy Scriptures regularly and systematically. He should betake himself to the company of the wise. He should practise right conduct, right thinking, right speaking and right acting. He should practise regular meditation. By and by all old vicious desires and sensual

cravings and evil propensities will vanish. Hey Saumya!
Lead a life of perfect contentment. Contentment is the bliss
of life. The cold ambrosial waters of contentment will
quickly extinguish the fire of desires. Contentment is the
chief sentinel who keeps watch over the domain of Peace or
the Kingdom of God.

The old subdued desires recur, persist and resist. They
assert: "O ungrateful man! You gave me shelter in your
mind all along. You enjoyed various objects of the world
through me only. If there is no desire for food and drink,
how can you enjoy food and drink? If there is no desire for
sexual union, how can you enjoy a woman? Why are you so
cruel towards me now? I have every right to dwell in this
abode of your mind. Do whatever you like." But you should
not be discouraged even a bit by these threats. All desires.
will be thinned out gradually by meditation and Yoga. They
will eventually perish in toto beyond resurrection.

A strong mind has influence over a weak mind. Mind
has influence over the physical body. Mind acts upon
matter. Mind brings bondage. Mind gives you liberation.
Mind is the devil. Mind is your best friend. Mind is your
Guru (Spiritual Preceptor). You will have to tame your
mind. You will have to discipline your mind. You will have
to control your mind. This is all you have to do.

Study your feelings and emotions. Analyse them.
Dissect them. Do not identify yourself with these feelings
and emotions. Separate yourself from these feelings and
emotions. Stand as a silent witness. Identification with these
feelings and emotions is the cause of bondage and misery.

Anger is a modification of desire in the mind. There is no modification in the Self or the real "I" or Atman. A worldly man identifies himself with anger and so he becomes miserable. This is ignorance only. The body and the mind are your instruments for growth and evolution. Identify yourself with the big, infinite "I" by utilising these two instruments and become a master of your mind and body. You are the driver of this engine—body and mind. Assert your birthright and become free, my child. Understand the trick of this mischievous mind. It has played with you long enough. Attain complete mastery over it. You can do this easily by the practice of Yoga.

Watch and chop and clip the thoughts as soon as they arise from the mind. Kill them dead on the spot. If you find it difficult to do this, become indifferent. Do not mind them. Allow them to take their own shape. They will soon die by themselves. Or, sometimes you can chop the thoughts and when you get tired of doing so, you can adopt the method of remaining indifferent. The latter method is more easy. If you tie a monkey to a post, it becomes more turbulent; if you allow it to move about at its own will and pleasure, it is not so very turbulent. Even so, when you try to fix the mind at a point, it becomes more turbulent. Therefore various kinds of evil thoughts enter into the minds of neophytes at the time of concentration. But they need not be unnecessarily alarmed. If you find it difficult to focus the mind at one point, allow it to jump a while like a monkey. Do not wrestle with the mind. It will soon get exhausted and will then be waiting to obey your behests. Now you can tackle it easily.

Free yourself from the tyranny of the mind. It has tormented you mercilessly for so long a time. You have allowed it to indulge in sensual pleasures and have its own ways. Now is the time to curb it just as you would curb a wild horse. Be patient and persevering. Practise daily thoughtlessness or inhibition of thoughts. The task may be difficult in the beginning. It will be indeed disgusting and tiring, but the reward is great. You will reap Immortality, Supreme Joy, Eternal Peace and Infinite Bliss. Therefore practise diligently in right earnest. It is worth doing. Be on the alert. If you are sincere in your wish and strong in your resolve, nothing is impossible under the sun to accomplish. Nothing can stand in your way. If you fail in your attempt, do not be discouraged. Remember the thrilling story of the dreadful fight between Hercules and the prodigious giant. In the course of his journey in quest of adventures, Hercules encountered a monster, who was so wonderfully contrived by nature that every time he touched the earth, he became ten times as strong as before. By remembering this incident you will get inner strength and courage. You are bound to succeed.

Realise that you are neither body nor mind, that you were never born nor will you ever die, that you are invincible, that nothing in this world can hurt you, that you are the Sun around whom the whole universe revolves. The whole knowledge is treasured up within the chambers of your heart. Procure the key and unlock the doors of Knowledge. Yoga is the Key. You will attain unruffled peace, marvellous self-control and tremendous will-power.

Behold! There on the banks of the holy Ganga at Rishikesh, Himalayas, a Sage, a Paramahamsa Sannyasin of eighty summers, with lustrous eyes, serene face, magnetic personslity, bright complexion sits with a loin-cloth only. There is a small grass-hut beside him underneath a tree. Inside the hut you will find a small wooden bowl (Kamandalu) for keeping water and an ordinary stick. This is all his personal effect. He is always sitting there in a contemplative mood. He never talks, nor laughs, but occasionally nods his roundshapely head and smiles gently. He never stirs from the place. He is unaffected by the heat of the summer sun or the biting cold of the winter. He never uses blankets, no, not even in winter. What a wonderful power of endurance! He lives on some milk and fruits only. His heart is filled with purity, mercy, compassion, sympathy and love!

People from various parts of the country flock to him in hundreds and thousands in season and out of season with flowers and fruits in their hands, prostrate at his Holy Feet, worship him with their offerings and leave the place with his ready blessings. He never talks, but all doubts are cleared in his mere presence. People forget the world, their families, their children. They bathe in his magnetic aura. Such is the benign influence of a liberated sage who is verily a beacon-light to the world at large.

Now here is a man living in the busiest part of a metropolis. He earns a fat salary. He spends half of his earnings in gambling and in drinking The other half goes to cinema and prostitutes. He eats fish, meat and smokes heavily. He runs into debts every month and finds it hard to make both ends meet. He dislikes sages and saints. He has no faith in God or in scriptures. He is very cruel-hearted. He attends ballrooms and theatres, goes to bed at 2 a.m. and gets up at 9 a.m. He wears a care-worn face even though he appears in costly silken finery. He is always gloomy and depressed. His heart is filled with lust, anger, greed, vanity, hypocrisy and egoism. Compare for a moment the life of this man with that of the magnanimous Sage of the Himalayas! They are poles asunder. The one is a God-man, the other is a bruteman. But if the brute-man seeks the company of the God-man, he will surely give up his old dirty habits. Just as iron is transmuted into gold by the touch of the philosopher's stone, so also the brute-man will be radically changed into a veritable saint by and by through constant contact with a developed Yogi.

Good friend! Slay this serpent of ignorance mercilessly. Get Knowledge of Self. This will give your Freedom or Liberation. Ignorance is your deadliest enemy. He has plundered the Jewel of Wisdom for long ages. Rise above temptations of this little world. This world is a show for five minutes directed by the juggler, Maya or mind. Beware. Do not get yourself entrapped. Money, woman, power, name, fame,—these are the five tempting baits of Maya. These who have not fallen victims to these illusory baits will surely reach the other shore of immortality and fearlessness—the shore beyond darkness, where there is perennial joy and eternal sunshine. Reach this shore through indefatigable struggle, rigid discipline and rigorous practice of Yoga.

From the condition of your mind, from your feelings and conduct, you can very well understand the nature of your actions in your previous lives and can nullify or counteract the effects of evil actions by doing good actions, Tapas, discipline and meditation. Try to lead a life of non-attachment. Discipline your mind carefully. No one is free from pains, diseases, troubles, difficulties. You will have to rest in your divine nature. Then alone you will draw strength to face the difficulties of life. Then only you will have a balanced mind. Then only you will not be affected by external morbid influences and discordant vibrations. Regular meditation in the morning will give you new strength and inner life of joy and bliss. Practise meditation. Feel this joy and bliss despite your stormy conditions and adverse circumstances. Gradually you will grow spiritually. You will attain Self-realisation.

Abandon this eat-drink-and-be-merry policy. Look always upwards and onwards. Have an ideal before you. Live up to it at any cost. You can become as great as anyone else. Give up this inferiority-complex. Give up the superiority-complex also. The idea of inferiority and superiority is born of ignorance. Inferioritycomplex will cause worry. Superioritycomplex will generate pride and vanity. Put up the switch of the eternal Light in the innermost chambers of your heart. Keep the Divine Flame burning steadily. Feed it regularly. Throw your whole heart and soul in spiritual practices. Waste not even a single minute. Be persistent and methodical in your Sadhana. Marshal up all your forces properly and powerfully even as the Lieutenant-General in the army marshals up the armies on the battlefield. All miseries will melt away soon. You will shine as a glorious Jivanmukta with the highest realisation. All sense of separateness, distinction, duality, difference will vanish out of sight. You will feel oneness and unity everywhere. You will feel that there is nothing but Brahman or God. What a magnanimous vision you are blessed with! What an exalted state, what a sublime, soul-stirring and stupendous experience will be yours! You will get dumbfounded. This state is indescribable. You must experience it by direct intuitive perception.

Introspect daily in the morning and examine the various nooks and corners of your heart. The mind is very diplomatic and cunning. The ego will keep several desires for secret gratification. Many desires will be lurking in your mind. It is very hard to detect their presence. Aspirants who are puffed up with their scholarly erudition and some powers (Siddhis) cannot trace the existence of these under-currents of desires in their minds. They pose themselves as great Yogins, deliver lectures in various parts of the world, build Ashrams and make lady-disciples. Nevertheless, it should be admitted, their speeches do not produce any deep impression in the minds of the hearers. These speeches are like empty bullets. The secret desires attack the student of Yoga mercilessly, whenever a suitable opportunity presents itself and destroys all his noble qualities and sublime ideals. They pounce upon the student of Yoga with a vengeance and redoubled vigour and bring a hopeless downfall that has no parallel. Those who have a pure, subtle intellect, who remember God always, who thirst for communion with Him, who practise daily introspection, self-analysis and meditation will be able to detect the presence of lurking desires, not others. He who has abandoned all desires, who is free from all yearnings, attains everlasting Peace. He enjoys the supremest Happiness. The fewer the desires, the greater the happiness. That desireless Yogi who roams about in the world with a loin-cloth and a blanket only is the happiest man in all the three worlds.

Selfishness is a negative attribute of the lower mind. It is a modification of desire that arises in a mind filled with passion. It is the first-born child of ignorance or indiscrimination. It is the greatest obstacle to the practice of Yoga. It is the bane of life. It contracts the heart *ad infinitum* and intensifies the idea of separateness from others. Selfishness goes hand in hand with egoism, hypocrisy, vanity, miserliness. cunningness, dishonesty and pride.

How to eradicate this selfishness? The answer is simple enough. Selfless service in some form or another, cultivation of the opposite virtuous qualities, viz., nobility, magnanimity, disinterestedness, integrity, generosity, charitable nature, mercy and universal love—all these will pave a long way in the eradication of this dire malady, the deadly foe of peace and Yoga. Positive overpowers the negative. This is an infallible dictum in Yoga.

To sum up the fundamental requisites for the practice of Yoga: You should have absolute fearlessness, regard for every creature that breathes, respect for truth, continence, absence of greed, a life of contentment, austerity, absence of anger and hypocrisy. Moral excellence is not the final goal of life but is only the means to that end. When the Yogi is established in these virtues, he gets some powers such as effectiveness of speech, arrival of unsought wealth, vigour of body and mind, clear and lucid undertaking of life's events, clarity of thought, steadiness of attention, control of the senses, immense joy and intuition.

Beloved Immortal Self! Observe vow of silence. Keep the mind fully occupied. Sit on your favourite Asana and do regular meditation. Sing the Name of the Lord. Twirl the beads. Study the Scriptures. Practise celibacy or be very, very moderate in sexual acts. Take almonds and sugar-candy every morning.[7] Do not consult doctors. Do not think of your disease. Divert the mind from the body. Be cheerful always. Smile, whistle, laugh, dance in joy and ecstasy. Think of God and meditate upon Him with true devotion and feeling and merge in Him. This is the goal of life. You have attained it after a long and continued struggle for some years with zeal and enthusiasm. You have now become a Jivanmukta (living liberated soul). Hail, hail to thee, a thousand hails, my child'

---

7  *Soak ten or twelve almond-seeds overnight in cold water. Peel off the skin the next mornmg and eat them with sugar-candy.*

# YOGIC DIET

A diet that is wholly conducive to the practice of Yoga and spiritual progress is called Yogic diet. Diet has intimate connection with the mind. Mind is formed out of the subtlest portion of food. Sage Uddalaka instructs his son Svetaketu "Food, when consumed becomes threefold: the gross particles become excrement, the middling ones flesh and the fine ones the mind. My child, when curd is churned, its fine particles which rise upwards, form butter. Thus, my child, when food is consumed, the fine particles which rise upwards form the mind. Hence verily the mind is food." Again you will find in the Chhandogya Upanishad: "By the purity of food one becomes purified in his inner nature; by the purification of his inner nature he verily gets memory of the Self; and by the attainment of the memory of the Self, all ties and attachments are severed."

Diet is of three kinds viz., Sattvic diet, Rajasic diet and Tamasic diet. Milk, barely, wheat, cereals, butter, cheese, tomatoes, honey, dates, fruits, almonds and sugar-candy are all Sattvic foodstuffs. They render the mind pure and calm. Fish, eggs, meat, salt, chillies and asafoetida are Rajasic foodstuffs. They excite passion. Beef, wine, garlic, onions and tobacco are Tamasic foodstuffs. They fill the mind with anger, darkness and inertia.

Lord Krishna says to Arjuna: "The food which is dear to each is threefold. Hear the distinctions of these. The foods which increase vitality, energy, vigour, health and joy and which are delicious, bland, substantial and agreeable are dear to the pure. The passionate desire foods that are bitter, sour, saline, excessively hot, pungent, dry and burning and which produce pain, grief and disease. The food which is stale, tasteless, putrid and rotten, leavings and impure is dear to the Tamasic." (Bhagavad-Gita. Ch. VII-8, 9, 10).

Food plays an important part in meditation. Different foods produce different effects on different compartments of the brain. For purposes of meditation, the food should be light, nutritious and Sattvic. Milk, fruits, almonds, butter, sugar-candy, green gram, Bengal gram soaked in water overnight, bread, etc., are all very helpful in meditation. *Thed* (a kind of root available in abundance in the Himalayan regions) is very Sattvic. Tea and sugar should be used in moderation. It is better if you can give them up entirely. Dried ginger-powder can be mixed with milk and taken frequently. Indian Yogins like this very much. Another health-giving stuff is myrobalan of the yellow variety which can be chewed now and then. In the Vagbhata it is represented as even superior to a nourishing mother. It takes care of the body better than a mother does. A mother gets annoyed with her child sometimes, but myrobalan always keeps an even temperament and is cheerful and enthusiastic in attending to the well-being of human beings. It preserves semen and stops all nocturnal emissions. Potato, boiled without salt or baked on fire, is also an excellent food for practitioners.

A beginner should be careful in choosing food-stuffs of Sattvic nature. Food exercises tremendously vast influence over the mind. You can see it obviously in everyday-life. It is very difficult to control mind after a heavy, sumptuous, indigestible, rich meal. The mind runs, wanders and jumps like an ape all the time. Alcohol causes great excitement of the mind.

Evolution is better than revolution. You should not make sudden changes in anything, particularly so in matters pertaining to food and drink. Let the change be slow and gradual. The system should accommodate it without any trouble. *Nature non agit per saltum* (nataure never moves by leaps).

Food is only a mass of energy. Water and air also supply energy to the body. You can live without food for several days; but you cannot live without air even for a few minutes. Oxygen is even more important. What is wanted to feed the body is energy. If you can supply this energy by any other means, you can entirely dispense with food. Yogins live without food by drinking nectar. This nectar flows through a hole in the palate. It dribbles and nourishes the body. A Jnani can draw energy directly from his pure, irresistible will and support the body without any food whatsoever. If you know the process of drawing the energy from the Cosmic Energy, then you can maintain the body for any length of time and can dispense with food completely.

Food is of four kinds. There are liquids which are drunk; solids which are pulverised by the teeth and eaten; .there are semi-solids which are taken in by licking; and there are soft articles that are swallowed without mastication. All articles of food should be thoroughly masticated in the mouth until they are reduced to quite a liquid before being swallowed. Then only they can be readily digested, absorbed and assimilated in the system.

The diet should be such as can maintain physical efficiency and good health. The well-being of an individual depends more on perfect nutrition than on anything else. Various sorts of intestinal diseases, increased susceptibility to infectious diseases, lack of high vitality and power of resistance, rickets, scurvy, anaemia or poverty of blood, beriberi, etc., are due to faulty nutrition. It should be remembered that it is not so much the climate as food which plays the vital role in producing a strong healthy body or a weakling suffering from a host of diseases. An appreciable knowledge of the science of dietetics is essential for everybody, especially for spiritual aspirants, to keep up physical efficiency and good health. Aspirants should be able to make out a cheap and well-balanced diet from only a certain articles of diet. What is needed is a well-balanced diet, not a rich diet. A *rich* diet produces diseases of the liver, kidneys and pancreas. A well-balanced diet helps a man to grow, to turn out more work, increases his body-weight, and keeps up the efficiency, stamina and a high standard of vim and vigour. You are what you eat.

Where can Sannyasins in India, who live on public alms get a well-balanced diet? On some days they get pungent stuffs only, on some other days sweetmeats only and yet on some other days sour things only. But they are able to draw the requisite energy through power of meditation. This unique Yogic method is unknown to the medical profession and to the scientists. Whenever the mind is concentrated, a divine wave bathes all the tissues with a divine elixir. All the cells are renovated and vivified.

Gluttons and epicureans cannot dream of getting success in Yoga. He who takes moderate diet, who has regulated his diet can become a Yogi, not others. That is the reason why Lord Krishna says: "Verily Yoga is not for him who eateth too much, nor who abstaineth to excess, nor who is too much addicted to sleep, nor even to wakefulness, O Arjuna! Yoga killeth out all pain for him who is regulated in eating and amusement, regulated in performing actions, regulated in sleeping and waking." (Bhagavad-Gita: Ch. VI-16-17). Therefore take pleasant, wholesome and sweet food half-stomachful; fill a quarter stomach with water and allow the remaining quarter stomach free for expansion of gas. Offer up the act to the Lord. This is moderate diet.

All articles that are putrid, stale, decomposed, unclean, twice cooked, kept overnight, should be abandoned. The diet should be fresh, simple, light, bland, wholesome, easily digestible and nutritious. He who lives to eat is a sinner, but he who eats to live is verily a saint. In the Siva Samhita it is said: "Yoga should not be practised irnmediately after a meal, nor when one is very hungry; before beginning the practice, some milk and butter should be taken."

You will find in the Yoga-Tattva Upanishad: "The proficient in Yoga should abandon the food detrimental to the practice of Yoga. He should give up salt, mustard, sour things, hot, pungent or bitter articles, asafoetida, women, emaciation of the body by fasts etc. During the early stages of practice, food of milk and ghee is ordained; also food consisting of wheat, green pulse and red rice is said to favour the progress. Then he will be able to retain his breath as long as he likes. By thus retaining the breath as long as he likes, Kevala-Kumbhaka (cessation of breath without inhalation and exhalation) is attained. When Kevala-Kumbhaka is attained by one and thus inhalation and exhalation are dispensed with, there is nothing unattainable in the three worlds to him."

In the Bhikshuka-Upanishad you will find: "Paramahamsas like Samavartaka, Aruni, Svetaketu, Jada Bharata, Dattatreya, Suka, Vamadeva, Haritaki and others take eight mouthfuls and strive after Moksha alone through the path of Yoga."

Manu, Jesus and Buddha exhorted the people to refrain from using liquors, intoxicants and drugs as these are deleterious in their effects. No spiritual progress is possible without abandoning them.

The vast majority of persons dig their graves through their teeth. No rest is given to the stomach. After all, man wants very little on this bountiful earth—a few loaves of bread, a little butter and some cold water. This will amply suffice to keep the life going. People, on the contrary, stuff their stomachs with all sorts of things, eatable and uneatable, on account of the force of habit even when there is no appetite. This is very bad. All diseases take their origin in overloading the stomach. Hunger is the best sauce. If there is hunger, food can be digested well. If you have no appetite, do not take anything. Let the stomach enjoy a full holiday.

A variety of dishes overworks the stomach, induces capricious appetite and renders the tongue fastidious. Then it becomes difficult to please the tongue. Therefore control the tongue first; then all the other senses can be easily controlled.

Man has invented so many kinds of dishes just to satisfy his palate and has made life complex and miserable. He calls himself a civilised man, when he is really ignorant and deluded by the senses. His mind gets upset when he cannot get his usual dishes in a new place. Is this real strength? He has become an absolute slave of his tongue. This is very deplorable. Be natural and simple in eating and drinking. Moderation is Yoga. Eat to live and not live to eat. Follow this golden rule and be happy. You can then devote more time to Yoga practices.

A Yogic student who spends his time wholly in pure meditation wants very little food. One or one and a half seers of milk and some fruits per day will quite suffice. But a Yogi who ascends the platform for vigorous active work wants abundant nutritious food.

Vegetarian diet has been acclaimed to be most conducive to spiritual and psychic advancement. It has been found that meat augments animal passion and decreases intellectual capacity. While it is true that meat-eating countries are physically active and strong, the same cannot be said of their spiritual attainments. Meat is not at all necessary for the keeping up of perfect health, rigour and vitality. On the contrary, it is highly deleterious to health. It brings in its train a host of ailments such as tape-worm, albuminuria and other diseases of the kidneys. Killing of animals for food is a great sin. Instead of killing the egoism and the idea of "mine-ness," ignorant people kill innocent animals under pretext of sacrifice to goddess, but in reality it is meant to please their own tongue or palate. What inhuman horrible crimes are being committed in the name of God and Religion! Ahimsa (non-injuring) is the first virtue that a spiritual aspirant should try to possess. You should have reverence for life. Lord Jesus says: "Blessed are the merciful, for they shall obtain mercy." Mahavira shouted in a trumpet-like voice: "Regard every living being as thyself and harm no one." The Law of Karma is inexorable, unrelenting, immutable. The pain you inflict upon another will surely rebound upon you and the happiness you radiate will come back to you adding to your happiness. He who knows this Law will not hurt anybody.

Meat-eating and alcoholism are closely allied. The craving for liquor dies a natural death, when the meat is withdrawn. The question of birth-control becomes very difficult in the case of those who take meat. To them mind-control is next to impossible. Mark how the meat-eating tiger and the cow or elephant living on green grass are poles asunder! The one is wild and ferocious, the other is mild and peaceful. Meat has direct influence on the different compartments of the brain.

The first and foremost step in the spiritual advancement of an aspirant is the giving up of meat. The Divine Light will not descend, if the stomach is loaded with meat. In large meat-eating countries cancer mortality is very high. Vegetarians keep up sound health till old age. Even in the West doctors in hospitals put patients on a regimen of vegetable diet. They convalesce quickly. It is welcome sign to see that at least in some of the countries of Europe vegetarian hotels are springing up in amazing numbers, and it is not too much to expect that in the course of a decade or two the Westerners will become quite a different race of people altogether in their food, dress, manners, habits and social customs.

Pythagoras seems to bewail when he says: "Beware, O mortals, of defiling your bodies with sinful food. There are cereals, there are fruits bending their branches down by their weight, and luxurious grapes on the vines. There are sweet vegetables and herbs which the fire can render palatable and mellow. Nor are you denied milk, nor honey, fragrance of the aroma of the thyme flower. The bountiful earth offers you an abundance of pure food and provides for meals obtainable without slaughter and bloodshed."

Fasting is interdicted for practitioners of Yoga as it produces weakness. But occasional mild fasts are highly beneficial. They will overhaul the system thoroughly, give rest to the stomach and the intestines and eliminate uric acid. Yogic students may take one full meal at 11 o'clock, a cup of warm milk in the morning and half a seer of milk and some plantains (or oranges or apples) at night with much advantage. The night meal should be very light. If the stomach is overloaded, sleep will supervene and as too much sleep is injurious to Yogic practices, one cannot make any real headway in the path of Yoga. Therefore a diet consisting of milk and fruits alone is a splendid menu for all practitioners.

Aspirants should avoid all narcotics, coffee, tea, alcohol and smoke that stimulate the senses. Our senses are compared to restive horses, and they become uncontrollable by taking narcotics. You should control them by refraining from taking narcotics. We are all slaves of our senses more or less and the senses in turn are the slaves of narcotics. If you really crave for perfection, control of mind and success in Yoga, avoid these narcotics by all possible means.

Boil half a seer of milk along with some boiled rice, ghee and sugar. This is called *Charu*. This is an excellent food for Yogic practitioners. This is for dinner. Half a seer of milk and some fruits will do for the night. Try this prescription and tell me the benefits you have derived in your Sadhana.

Milk should not be boiled too much. It should be removed from fire the moment the boiling point is reached. Excessive boiling destroys all nutritious principles and vitamins and renders milk unfit for consumption. Milk is an ideal food for aspirants. It is a perfect food by itself.

Fruit-diet exercises a marvellous influence upon the constitution. This is a natural diet. Fruits are tremendous energy-producers. Fruits and milk help concentration and meditation. Barley, wheat, milk, ghee and honey promote longevity of life and increase power and stamina. Fruit-juice and the water wherein sugar-candy is dissolved are very good drinks. Butter mixed with sugar-candy and almonds soaked in water overnight will cool the system.

Above all do not make much fuss about your diet. You need not advertise to everyone that you are able to live on a particular form of diet. The observance of such Niyama (rules) is for your own advancement in the spiritual path and you will not be spiritually benefited by giving publicity to your practices. There are many nowadays who make it their profession to make money and their livelihood by performing some Yoga-Asanas, Pranayama or by having some diet regulation as eating only raw articles or leaves or roots. These people cannot have any real spiritual growth. The goal of life is Self-realisation, and aspirants should always keep this in view and do intense Sadhana with zeal and patience.

Live a natural simple life. Take simple food that is wholly agreeable to your system. You should have your own menu to suit your constitution. You are yourself the best judge to select a Sattvic diet. In the matter of food and drink you will do well to eat and drink as a master. You should not have the least craving for any particular diet. You should not become a slave to this food or that food. Simple, natural, non-stimulating, tissue-building, energy-producing, non-alcoholic food and drink will keep the mind calm and pure and will help the student of Yoga in his practices and in the attainment of the goal of life.

## TABLE SHOWING SATTVIC, RAJASIC AND TAMASIC ARTICLES OF DIET

| SATTVIC | RAJASIC | TAMASIC |
|---------|---------|---------|
| Cow's milk. | Fish. | Beef. |
| Cream. | Eggs. | Pork. |
| Cheese. | Meat. | Wine. |
| Butter. | Salt. | Onions. |

| | | |
|---|---|---|
| Curd. | Chillies. | Garlic. |
| Ghee. | Chutney. | Tobacco. |
| Sweet fruits. | Asafoetida. | Rotten things. |
| Apples. | Pickles. | Stale things. |
| Bananas. | Tamarind. | Unclean things. |
| Grapes. | Mustard. | Twice cooked |
| Papaya. | Sour things. | things. |
| Pomegranates. | Hot things. | All intoxicants. |
| Mangoes. | Tea. | All liquors. |
| Oranges. | Coffee. | All drugs. |
| Pears. | Cocoa. | |
| Pineapples. | Ovaltine. | |
| Guavas. | White sugar. | |
| Figs. | Carrots. | |
| Vegetables. | Turnips. | |
| Cocount. | Spices. | |
| Brinjals. | | |
| Potatoes. | | |
| Cabbages. | | |
| Spinach. | | |

Tomatoes. Cucumber. Pumpkin. Cauliflower. Lady's finger.
Peaches. Almonds. Pistachios. Raisins. Wheat. Red rice.
Unpolished rice. Barley. Oat-meal. Dried peas. Dates.
Sugar-candy. Green gram. Bengal gram. Green pulse.
Groundnut. Cereals. Dried ginger. Myrobalan. Lemon.
Honey. *Charu.*

## Lesson V

# OBSTACLES IN YOGA[8]

There are certain obstacles in the path of Yoga, which you should, by all means, overcome in the very beginning of your Yogic career. If you do not adequately guard yourself against these impediments in right time by the warning voice of your Guru, they will smash all your hopes and aspirations to pieces and will eventually bring about miserable downfall.

Lust, greed, anger, hatred, jealousy, fear, inertia, depression, prejudice, intolerance, evil company, arrogance, self-sufficiency, desire for name and fame, curiosity, building castles in the air and hypocrisy are foremost among these. You should ever introspect and watch your mind. You should take effective measures to remove these obstacles root and branch.

"Women, beds, seats, dresses, and riches are obstacles in Yoga. Betels, dainty dishes, carriages, kingdoms, lordliness and powers; gold, silver, as well as copper, gems, aloe wood, and kine; learning the Vedas and the Sastras; dancing, singing and ornaments; harp, flute, and drum; riding on elephants and horses; wives and children, worldly

---

8 *A lecture delivered in the Willoughby Memorial Hall, Lakshmipur, by Swami Sivananda Sarasvati, on December 15, 1932*

enjoyments; all these are so many impediments." (Siva Samhita: Ch. V-3).

The Yogic student should not possess much wealth as it will drag him to worldly temptations. He may keep a small sum to get the wants of the body. Economical independence is of paramount importance to an aspirant; because it will relieve him from anxieties and will enable him to continue his practices uninterruptedly.

If you get easily offended even for trifling things, know that you cannot make any progress in Yoga and meditation. You should, hence, cultivate amiable, loving nature and adaptability. Some aspirants easily get offended, if their defects and vices are pointed out. They become indignant and begin to fight with the person who shows the defects. They think that the person is concocting them out of jealousy and hatred. This is bad. Others can very easily detect your defects. If you have no life of introspection, if your mind is of outgoing tendencies, how can you find out your own defects? Your self-conceit veils and blurs your mental vision. If you, therefore, want to grow in spirituality and Yoga, you must admit your defects, when they are pointed out by others. You must endeavour to eradicate them and must be really grateful to the man for pointing out your defects.

It is rather a difficult business to eradicate the self-assertive nature. This nature is born of ignorance only. Everyone has built his personality from beginningless time. This personality has grown very strong. It is hard to bend this personality and make it pliable and elstic. You want to dominate over others. You do not want to hear the opinions and arguments of others, even though they are quite logical, sound and tenable. You have a pair of jaundiced eyes. You say: "Whatever I say is correct. Whatever I do is correct. The views and actions of others are incorrect." You never admit your mistakes. You try your best to support your own whimsical views by crooked arguments. If arguments fail, you will take to vituperation and hand-to-hand fight also. If people fail to show you respect and honour, you are instantauleously thrown into a fit of fury. You are immensely pleased with anybody who begins to flatter you. You will tell any number of lies to justify yourself. Self-justification goes hand in hand with self-assertive Rajasic nature. You can never grow in Yoga so long as you have this self-assertive nature with the habit of self-justification. You should change your mental attitude. You must develop the habit of looking at matters from the view-point of others. You must have the new vision of righteousness and truthfulness. Then alone you will grow in Yoga and spirituality. You should treat respect and honour as offal and poison, and censure and dishonour as ornament and nectar.

You will also find it hard to adjust yourself to the ways and habits of others. Your mind is filled, as it were, with likes and dislikes, prejudice of caste, creed and colour. You are quite intolerant. The faultfinding nature is ingrained in you. You jump at once to find the faults of others. You cannot see the good in others; you have a pair of morbid eyes. You cannot appreciate the meritorious actions of others. You brag of your own abilities and merits. That is the reason why you fight with all people and cannot maintain cordial relations with others for long time. You should overcome these defects by developing tolerance, love and other good virtues.

The old Samskaras (latent impressions) of vanity, cunningness, crookedness, arrogance, petty-mindedness, fighting, boasting or bragging nature, self-esteem or thinking too much of yourself, speaking ill of others, belittling others may be still lurking in your mind. You can never shine until you remove these faults thoroughly. Success in Yoga is not possible unless these undesirable negative qualities of lower nature are completely eradicated.

Those who engage themselves in hot discussions, vain debates, wranglings, lingual warfare and intellectual gymnastics cause serious damage to their astral bodies. Much energy is wasted. The astral body gets actually inflamed and an open sore is formed. Blood becomes hot. It bubbles like milk over fire. Ignorant people have no idea of the disastrous effects of unnecessary hot discussions and argumentations. Those who are in the habit of arguing unnecessarily and entering into vain discussions cannot expect an iota of progress in Yoga. Aspirants must entirely give up unnecessary discussions. They should destroy the impulses by careful introspection.

You have heard several brilliant lectures, delivered by learned monks or Sannyasins. You have listened to several discourses and expositions on the Bhagavad-Gita, the Ramayana, the Bhagavata and the Upanishads. You have also heard several valuable moral and spiritual instructions. But you have not at all endeavoured to put anything into serious earnest practice and to do protracted solid Sadhana.

Mere intellectual assent to a religious idea, a little closing of the eyes in the morning and at night just to deceive yourself and the Indweller and the Witness, a little endeavour to stick to the daily spirtiual routine and to develop some virtues in a half-hearted, careless manner, some mild effort to carry out the instructions of your spiritual preceptor perfunctorily will not suffice. This kind of mentality should be entirely given up. You should follow the instructions of your master and the teachings of the Scriptures to the very letter. No leniency to the mind. There can be no half measures in the path of Yoga. Exact implicit and strict obedienee to the instructions is what is expected of you.

Do not make any thoughtless remarks. Do not speak even a single idle word. Give up idle talk, tall talk, big talk, loose talk. Avoid evil company. Become silent. Do not assert for rights in this physical, illusory plane. Do not fight for rights. Think more about your duties and less about your rights. These rights are worthless. Assert your birthright of God-consciousness. Then you are a wise man.

If you are endowed with good character, celibacy (Brahmacharya), truthfulness, mercy, love, tolerance, forgiveness, serenity, these qualities will more than counterbalance many other evil qualities you may possess. Then gradually these evil qualities also will vanish, if you are careful, if you focuss your attention on them.

If you remain in the company of a developed saint, you will be really benefited by his magnetic aura and wonderful spiritual currents. His company will be like a fortress for you. You will not be affected by evil influences. There is no fear of downfall. You can have rapid spiritual progress.

Young aspirants should remain in the company of their Gurus or other experienced saints till they are firmly moulded and established in deep meditation. Nowadays many young aspirants wander aimlessly from place to place. They do not care to hear the instructions of their masters. They want independence from the very start. Hence they do not make any progress in Yoga.

Humour is a rare gift of nature. It helps aspirants in their march on the spiritual path. It removes depression. It keeps one cheerful. It brings joy and mirth. But you should not cut jokes at the expense of others and wound their feelings. The humorous words must educate and correct others.

You should laugh in a mild, delicate and decent manner. Silly giggling, guffaw, or boisterous, indecent, unrefined laughter in a rude manner should be given up, because it prevents the spiritual progress and destroys serenity of mind and serious magnanimous attitude. Sages smile through their eyes. It is grand and thrilling. Intelligent aspirants only can understand this. Don't be childish and silly.

Even the slight annoyance and irritability affect the mind and the astral body. You should not allow these evil modifications (Vrittis) to manifest in the mind-lake. They may burst out as big waves of anger at any moment, if you are weak and careless. They should be nipped in the bud. You should develop the noble qualities of forgiveness, love and sympathy for others. There should not be the least disturbance in the mind-lake. It should be perfectly calm and serene. Then only meditation is possible.

Success in Yoga is possible only if the aspirant practises profound and constant meditation. He must practise self-restraint at all times, because all of a sudden the senses may become turbulent. That is the reason why Lord Krishna says to Arjuna: "O son of Kunti! The excited senses of even a wise man, though he be striving impetuously, carry away his mind. For the mind, which follows in the wake of the wandering senses, carries away his discrimination, as the wind (carries away) a boat on the waters." (Bhagavad-Gita: Ch. II-60, 67).

A terrible fit of anger shatters the physical nervous system and produces a deep and lasting impression on the astral body. Dark arrows will shoot forth from the astral body. The germs that caused the epidemic of Spanish flu may die, but the wave of influenza still continues in various parts for a long time. Even so, though the effect of the fit of anger in the mind may subside in a short time, the vibration or wave continues to exist for days or weeks together in the astral body. Slight, unpleasant feeling that lasts in the mind for five minutes may produce vibration in the astral body for two or three days. A terrible fit of wrath will produce deep inflammation of the astral body. An open sore will be formed on the surface of the astral body. It will take months for the healing of the ulcer. Have you now realised the serious consequences of anger? Do not fall a victim to anger. Control it by forgiveness, love, mercy, sympathy, enquiry (of "who am I?") and consideration for others.

Worry, depression, unholy thoughts and hatred produce a kind of crust or dark layer on the surface of the mind or astral body. This crust or rust or dirt prevents the beneficial influences to get entry inside, but it allows the evil forces or lower influences to operate. Worry does great harm to the astral body and the mind. Energy is wasted by this worry-habit. Nothing is gained by worrying. It causes inflammation of the astral body and drains the vitality of man. It should be eradicated by the practice of cheerfulness, vigilant introspection and keeping the mind fully occupied.

By continence, devotion to Guru and steady practice, success in Yoga comes after a long time. You should be patient and persevering.

Aspirants who take to seclusion generally become lazy after some time, as they do not know how to utilise their mental energy, as they do not have any daily routine, as they do not follow the instructions of their Gurus. They get Vairagya (dispassion and disgust for worldly enjoyments) in the beginning, but as they have no experience in the spiritual line, the Vairagya begins to wane. They do not make any real progress in the end. Intense and constant practice of Yoga is necessary for entering into Asamprajnata Samadhi.

If the Yogic student who practises meditation is gloomy, depressed and weak, surely there is some error in his Sadhana somewhere. True meditation makes the aspirant strong, cheerful and healthy. If the aspirants themselves are gloomy and peevish, how are they going to impart joy, peace and strength to others?

You will have to master every step in Yoga. Do not take up any higher step before completely mastering the lower step. Gradually ascend the successive stages boldly and cheerfully. This is the right royal road to perfection in Yoga.

Aspirants do not possess true and unshakable faith in their Gurus and the teachings of the Scriptures. Hence they fail to attain success in Yoga.

Sleepless vigilance is necessary, if you wish to· have rapid spiritual advancement. Never rest contented with a little achievement or success in the path, a little serenity of mind, a little one-pointedness of mind, some visions of angels and Devatas, a little faculty of thought-reading, and so on. There are still higher summits to ascend, higher regions to climb.

A Yogi claims that he can attain extraordinary powers and knowledge by subduing the passions and appetites and by practising Yama, Niyama and Yogic Samyama (concentration, meditation and Samadhi at one and the same time). Patanjali clearly warns the students that they should not be carried away by the temptations of powers. The gods themselves tempt the unwary Yogi by offering him a position similar to theirs. Aspirants run more after Siddhis (psychic powers) than after real spiritual attainment despite the clear note of warning.

Desire for powers will act like puffs of air which may blow out the lamp of Yoga that is being carefully fed. Any slackness in feeding it due to carelessness or selfishness will blow out the little spiritual lamp the Yogi has lighted after so much struggle and will hurl him down into the deep abyss of ignorance. He cannot rise up again to the original height to which he had ascended. Temptations are simply waiting to overwhelm the unwary aspirant or Yogi. Temptations of the astral, mental and the Gandharva worlds are more powerful than earthly temptations.

Patanjali enumerates the following nine obstacles: Disease, languor, doubt, carelessness, laziness, sensuality, mistaken notion, (false knowledge) tossing of mind and instability to remain in the state of Samadhi. He prescribes practice of concentration on one subject (Eka-Tattvabhyasa) to overcome them. This will give the aspirant steadiness and real inner strength. He further advocates the practice of friendship between equals, mercy towards inferiors, complacency towards superiors and indifference towards wicked people. This practice will generate peace of mind or composure and will destroy hatred, jealousy, etc. A new life will dawn in him, when he practises these virtues. Perseverance is needed. It is the key-note to success in Yoga. The Yogi is amply rewarded, when he gets full control over his mind. He enjoys the highest bliss of Asamprajnata Samadhi.

In the Yoga-Kundalini Upanishad you will find: "Diseases are generated in one's body through the following causes viz., sleeping in the day-time, late vigils overnight, excess of sexual intercourse, moving in crowds, the checking of the urine and the faeces, the evil of unwholesome food and laborious mental operations with Prana. If a Yogi is afraid of such diseases (when attacked by them), he says: "My diseases have arisen from the practice of Yoga." Then he will discontinue his practice. This is said to be the first obstacle. The second obstacle is doubt, the third carelessness, the fourth laziness, the fifth sleep, the sixth not leaving of objects (of sense), the seventh erroneous perception, the eighth sensual objects, the ninth want of faith and the tenth the failure to attain the truth of Yoga. A wise man should abandon these ten obstacles after great deliberation.

Fatigue is harmful for aspirants. They should avoid long walks and much exertion. When the state of tranquillity prevails during meditation, do not disturb the mind. Do not get up from your seat. Try to prolong the meditation.

You cannot please the world. Remember the story of the old man, his son and the donkey. Stick to your ideals, convictions and principles tenaciously, whether you become popular or unpopular, even if the whole world opposes you. Stand up boldly on your own principles of right conduct and right living. Do not retrace your steps even a fraction of an inch.

Do not dig shallow pits here and there for getting water. The pits will dry up soon. Dig a deep pit in one place. Centralise all your efforts here. You will get good water throughout the year. Even so, try to imbibe the spiritual teachings from one preceptor only. Drink deep from one man only. Sit at his feet for some years. There is no use of wandering from place to place, from one man to another man out of curiosity, losing faith in a short time. Do not have the everchanging mind of a prostitute. Follow the spiritual instructions of one man only. If you go to several people and follow their instructions, you will be bewildered. You will be in a dilemma.

Do not relax your efforts. Keep the Divine Flame burning steadily. You are nearing the goal. Thy light has come. There is Brahmic aura in your face. You have crossed many peaks and insurmountable summits in the spiritual path by dint of Untiring patient Sadhana. It is highly creditable indeed! You have made marvellous progress. I am highly pleased with you, O John! You will have to ascend one more peak and go through one more narrow pass. This demands some more patient effort and strength. You will have to melt your Sattvic egoism also. You will have to transcend the blissful state of Savikalpa Samadhi. The Brahmakara Vritti also should die. Then alone you will attain Bhuma, the highest goal of life. You can do this also. I am quite confident.

There at the summit of the Hill of Eternal Bliss, you can see now the Jivanmukta or the full-blown Yogi. He has climbed the stupendous heights through intense and constant struggle. He did severe rigorous spiritual Sadhana. He did profound meditation. He spent sleepless nights. He kept long vigils at night on countless occasions. He gradually ascended the heights step by step. He took rest at several halting-places. He persevered with patience and diligence. He surmounted many obstacles. He conquered despair, gloom and depression. Today he is a beacon-light to the world at large. You can also ascend to that summit, if only you will.[9]

---

9 *For further particulars vide my book "Sure Ways for Success in Life and God-realisation."*

# YOGA-ASANAS[10]

How many of you, sisters and brothers, find in yourselves the unmistakable signs of disease, declining health, vim, vigour and vitality? How many of you, may I ask again, feel actually the grip of premature old age? Why do you unjustly throw the whole blame on heredity without for a moment realising that for nearly thirty or thirty-five years you have been flouting the laws of life? Thirty-five years of wrong living! Thirty-five years of wrong feeding! Thirty-five years of wrong breathing! Thirty-five years of wrong thinking! Thirty-five years spent in abject ignorance of the relationship between brain and brawn! Thirtyfive years, in fact, spent in doing everything possible to develop the disease of "Old Age! "

Now suppose the whole situation is reversed, and in place of wrong living, wrong feeding, wrong breathing, etc., there is introduced right living, right feeding, right breathing, and so forth, what will be the effect? Will physical and mental degeneration give place to physical and mental regeneration? The answer given by the Seers of the East is an emphatic "YES". The Indian Yogins have

---

10For full detailed particulars vide my book "*Yoga Asanas.*"

conclusively proved that by following a regimen it is quite possible to rebuild the human body, to reconstruct the human mind, to regain lost youth, strength and beauty. The key to accomplish this remarkable feat according to the Saints, Sages and Rishis of yore is to be found in Yoga-Asanas.

You know what the word 'Yoga' means. It is union of the individual soul (Jivatman) with the Supreme Soul (Paramatman). Asana is an easy and comfortable seat or pose or posture. Thus the term Yoga-Asanas means certain postures by assuming any one of which the individual soul is united with the Supreme Soul quite easily by the Yogic practitioner. The relationship between mind and body is so complete and so subtle that it is no wonder that certain physical training will induce certain mental transformations.

A good many of you might have come across several persons capable of demonstrating these Yoga-Asanas some of which may seem at first sight disgusting and tiring. At any rate such persons are not uncommon in India. Some of my own students who are specialists in this branch of Yoga can do the various exercises with amazing grace and finish. It is wrong to suppose that these Yoga-Asanas are merely physical exercises founded by the ancient Rishis of India just as so many systems of physical culture have cropped up now both in Europe and in America. There is something spiritual, something divine at the bottom of this system for it awakens the sleeping Kundalini-Shakti, helps the Yogic student a lot in establishing himself fully in meditation and finally makes him taste the nectar of Cosmic Consciousness.

It is important to know what an ideal system of physical culture should be, so that you will be able to judge for yourself the value of Yoga-Asanas in the light of the ideal. That system can be safely said to be an ideal system which requires the smallest amount of energy to be spent in order to secure the greatest amount of benefit; which can effect a maximum increase in the vital index; which can build up a healthy nervous system; which can ensure health for the excretory organs of the body; which can take care of the circulatory system; and which can also develop the muscular system. Let us now see how far these few conditions are fulfilled by Yoga-Asanas.

Let me now prescribe a short but complete course of Yoga-Asanas which is more than sufficient for an average man (or woman) of health not only to maintain a high standard of health but also to achieve true success in Yoga. Yogic physical culture is only a means to an end, and not an end in itself. You need not, therefore, attach undue importance to this branch of Yoga alone to the gross neglect of the others. All the Asanas mentioned and illustrated in this book can be successfully practised without the personal contact of a teacher. Thousands are benefited in various ways by regularly practising these Asanas. The various exercises given in this book have been so arranged that strict adherence is expected of you. All Asanas should be done *invariably in the morning,* and not in the evening as you will find in some books on the subject. The reason for this emphasis is that in the evening everybody is tired of a day's work and as such will not be able to do the various exercises with a feeling of exhilaration and freshness which he or she would otherwise feel in the morning. There should absolutely be no feeling of depression or fatigue either before or during the performance of these exercises. This is an important point to remember, if you wish to enjoy the benefits of these exercises in the fullest measure. You need not go through the whole course everyday, but you must by all means be regular and systematic in the very little that you do, and be a master of all the exercises given in this book. Another point to remember is that the amount of energy expended in these exercises should on no account strain your system. Those of you who wish to do muscular exercises may do so in the evening. All Yóga-Asanas must be done on an empty stomach; but there is no harm if a small cup of milk, light tea or coffee is taken before commencing the exercises.

Asana is the third limb (Anga) of Yoga. If you are firmly established in Asanas, you will not feel the body at all. When you do not feel the body, qualities of the pairs of opposites will not affect you. When you are free from the effect of the pairs of opposites such as heat and cold, pleasure and pain, you will be able to take up the next higher step viz., Pranayama and practise it with an unruffled mind. Therefore you should select that posture which is easy and comfortable and in which you can remain long, say, three hours. Lord Krishna says: "Having in a cleanly spot established a firm seat, neither too high nor too low with cloth, skin, and *Kusa* grass thereon: making the mind one-pointed, with the actions of the mind and the senses controlled, let him, seated there on the seat, practise Yoga for the purification of the self. Holding erect and still the body, head and neck, firm, gazing at the tip of the nose, without looking around, serene-minded, fearless, firm in the vow of godly life, having restrained the mind, thinking on Me, and balanced, let him sit, looking up to Me as the Supreme." (Bhagavad-Gita: Ch. VI-11, 12 13).

Yoga aims at developing, will-power. A man of strong and dynamic will-power will always sit upright and walk with his chest thrown in front of his head; but a weak-willed person will change his posture often and often, while sitting or standing, will walk in a zigzag fashion, betraying infirmity and want of resolution of mind in every step. The practice of Asanas is of vital importance, and though the practice may be found to be painful and troublesome at the outset, when once the habit of sitting on one Asana for a considerable length of time is formed, you will feel a peculiar thrill and pleasure while seated there, and you will not like to change the pose on any account.

According to Patanjali Maharshi posture is that which is firm and comfortable. He does not lay any special stress on either Asana or Pranayama. It was only later on that the Hatha-Yogins developed these two limbs of Yoga, and, no doubt, they are of tremendous help to the Yogic student. While the Hatha-Yogins aim at the control and culture of the body, the Raja-Yogins aim at the control and culture of the mind. And as body and mind are interdependent, physical culture is *a sine qua non* to mental culture.

It is wrong to suppose that Yoga-Asanas are purely meant for the Indians and that they are ideally suited to Indian conditions. That it is not the case is proved by the following few instances. Mr. Harry Dikman, the Director-Founder of the Yoga Centre in Riga, Latvia (Europe) is a good specialist in these Yoga-Asanas,

Bandhas and Mudras and his opinion and advice to persons suffering from various kinds of diseases, curable and incurable, are increasingly becoming popular in Europe. I have not heard of another man either in Europe or in America, who takes such a keen and lively interest in this subject and is making researches in the same. You will be surprised to know that Mr. Harry Dikman is essentially a philosopher and a sage.

In California (U.S.A.) a young girl of about two and twenty, weighing, 280 lbs., due to much adiposity and therefore feeling completely dejected and forlorn, finally took recourse to Yoga-Asanas on the recommendation of a friend of hers, and in the course of six months time, to the astonishment and wonder of all, was able to reduce her body-weight to 180 lbs., by following the instructions of a specialist! The photographs of the girl taken before, during and after the six months course were lavishly published in various American journals and high tributes paid to the remarkable efficacy of Yoga-Asanas as the means of building up a radiant and healthy body and eradicating all kinds of diseases.

Mr Ernest Haekel of Los Angeles, California, Mr. Boris Sacharow of Berlin and several others interested in acquiring psychic powers by awakening the Kundalini are all instances to prove that Yoga-Asanas can be practised and are intended not only for India and the Indians but for the whole world and the humanity at large.

Practise either Padmasana or Siddhasana for meditative purposes, and the various other Asanas,

Bandhas, etc., for maintaining, a high standard of health, vigour, strength, vitality, and for keeping up Brahmacharya.

## (1) PADMASANA
### (THE LOTUS POSE)

Amongst the various poses prescribed for meditation, Padmasana is unique and foremost. It holds a very conspicuous place in the Yoga practices because great Rishis like Sandilya, Gheranda and several others have spoken of it in glowing terms. It is called Padmasana because of its full pose lending one the appearance of a full-blown lotus.

Sit on the .seat prescribed by Lord Krishna in the Bhagavad-Gita: Ch. VI-11. Stretch the legs forward, place the right foot gently at the left hip-joint, and the left foot similarly at the right hip-joint. Keep the spine erect. Place the right hand on the right knee-joint and the left hand on the left knee-joint.[11] Gaze gently at the tip of the nose. This is Padmasana. Practise this Asana for 5 minutes to start with and gradually increase the time to 3 hours. Padmasana destroys all diseases and bestows quick emancipation to the practitioner.

---

11 *Or you can make a finger-lock and keep the locked hands on the left heel. This is comfortable for some persons. Or you can place the right hand on the right knee-joint with palm facing upwards and the index finger touching the middle of the thumb; the left hand also should be placed on the left knee-joint with the palm facing upwards and the index finger touching the middle of the thumb in a similar manner.*

## (2) SIDDHASANA
### (THE PERFECT POSE)

Siddhasana is next to Padmasana in importance. Some eulogise it as even superior to Padmasana from the point of view of meditation. The Asana is so called because it is capable of giving the practitioner all Siddhis (psychic powers). Moreover it was and is the favourable pose of several Adepts in Yoga (Siddhas) .

Sit again on the seat prescribed by Lord Krishna as before. Stretch the legs forward. Place the left heel carefully at the anal aperture and the other heel on the root of the generative organ. Fix the chin on the chest. Gently gaze at the space between the two eyebrows without in any way straining your eyes.[12] Keep the spine erect. You can keep the hands and fingers just as in Padmasana. Start doing this for 5 minutes and slowly increase it to 3 hours. Young aspirants who wish to get themselves established in Brahmacharya should practise this Asana. "Through this posture the Yogi, leaving the world, attains the highest end and throughout the world there is no posture more sacred than this. By assuming and contemplating in this posture, the Yogi is freed from sin." (Siva-Samhita: Ch. III-87). Persons suffering, from syphilis, spermatorrhoea, piles,

---

12 *This is known as the Frontal Gaze. Take particular care not to strain your eye in any manner. Gaze very, very gently. If you find it difficult to do this also, simply close your eyes and concentrate on the heart-lotus or the space between the two eye-brows. This practice is doubly beneficial. It will not only not strain your eyes, but will also protect them from the risk of some foreign matter getting into them and causing unnecessary eye-trouble.*

diabetes and gonorrhoea will be greatly benefited by assuming this pose regularly for some time.

## (3)  SIRSHASANA
### (THE TOPSY-TURVY POSE)

This is called Sirshasana as you have to stand on the head. It is considered to be the king of all Asanas.

Spread a fourfold blanket. Squat on the ground and prepare a finger-lock by knitting the fingers of both the hands together. Make a convenient angle with the forearms. Let the finger-lock serve the purpose of a vertex. Keep the top of the head on the vertex. Slowly raise the lower part of the trunk, and then the legs. Now the whole body will stand at right angle with the ground. Remain in this pose for 5 seconds in the beginning and slowly increase the time to half an hour. Let the breathing be normal throughout. Bring the legs again slowly down without making any sudden jerk. Relax the body. This is important.

Sirshasana is a panacea for all human ills. It is extremely useful in keeping up Brahmacharya because the seminal energy is transmuted into Ojas-Sakti and stored up in the brain. This is sex-sublimation. Persons suffering from diseases of the eye, nose, head, throat, stomach, genito-urinary system, liver, spleen, lungs, renal colic, deafness, piles, asthma, consumption, pyorrhoea, constipation, and many other troubles will find great relief by its practice. Grey hairs and wrinkles will disappear. It augments the digestive fire and increases appetite. Ladies also can do this Asana. Sterility vanishes. Many uterine and ovarine diseases are cured. Indeed Sirshasana is a blessing and a gift to humanity. During the practice of this Asana the brain draws plenty of blood and energy. Memory increases wonderfully. Pt. Jawaharlal Nehru, the Prime Minister of India, was an ardent votary of Sirshasana. He managed to practise this pose daily somehow or other.

## (4)SARVANGASANA
### (ALL-MEMBERS POSE)

The next is Sarvangasana. It is so called because all parts of the body function during its performance.

Spread a thick blanket on the ground. Lie flat on your back. Then slowly raise the legs up, lifting the trunk and the hips vertically. Let the two hands support the back at the hips. Let the elbows rest on the ground. Form a chin-lock by firmly pressing the chin against the chest. In this posture the hinder part of the neck lies on the ground, and the trunk and legs stand in a straight line. Concentrate the mind at the thyroid gland that is situated at the root of the neck. Do this for 2 minutes to start with and increase the time to half an hour. Let the breathing be normal during the whole process.

Sarvangasana will build for you a healthy thyroid. A healthy thyroid means healthy functioning of all organs of the body. This pose centralises the blood in the spinal column and feeds it abundantly. It keeps the spine strong and elastic. You will have everlasting youth. It helps you not a little in keeping up Brahmacharya. It checks wet-dreams and rejuvenates the impotent. It is a blood and nervine tonic too. It removes dyspepsia, constipation and several other gastro-intestinal disorders. The benefits you derive from Sirshasana are also derived from Sarvangasana. A course of Sirsha-Sarvangasana will cure leprosy, powerfully rejuvenate the body and dispense with monkey-gland grafting.

## (5)  MATSYASANA
### (THE FISH POSE)

This pose is called Matsyasana because by assuming this posture and doing Plavini Pranayama you can float like the fish on water as long as you like.

Spread a thick blanket on the ground. Sit on it with legs fully stretched in front of you. Do Padmasana. Then lie flat on the back. Then resting the whole body on the elbows raise the trunk and head. Pressing the head well on the ground on the one side and the buttocks on the other, make an arch or a bridge of the trunk. Rest the hands on the thighs or catch hold of the toes, the right hand holding the left toe and the left hand the right toe.

Practise this Asana soon after Sarvangasana for one third of the time you devote to the latter, if you want the maximum benefits. Sarvangasana and Matsyasana go hand in hand. They must always be practised one after the other. When you have finished doing this Asana, slowly release the head with the help of the hands, sit erect and unlock the foot-lock.

Matsyasana gives a soothing massage to the neck and the shoulders. The stiffness of the neck is removed. Matsyasana helps deep breathing. The cervical and upper dorsal nerves are abundantly nourished with blood and toned up nicely. The endocrine, the pituitary and the pineal glands located in the brain are stimulated and toned. These glands play a vital part in the proper functioning of the various systems of the human body. Matsyasana is also the destroyer of many diseases. It cures constipation, asthma, consumption, chronic bronchitis, epilepsy, a certain type of obesity, the evil effects of masturbation, excessive sexual indulgence and waste of seminal powers, and is said to have cured leprosy also. It dispenses with the transplantation of monkey-thyroids to human beings for rejuvenation. Enlargement of the spleen is cured. Lost manhood, wasted vitality and misspent energy could be effectively regained by the assiduous practice of this posture. The heart is also massaged and you feel new and young.

## (6)BHUJANGASANA
### (THE COBRA POSE)

*Bhujanga* means a cobra in Sanskrit. This pose is called Bhujangasana because when the full pose is displayed, it lends one the appearance of a hooded cobra.

Spread a blanket on the ground. Lie on it face down and the muscles of the body completely relaxed. Place the palms on the ground just below the shoulders, bending them in the elbows. Touch the ground with the forehead and raise the head and the upper part of the body slowly just as a cobra raises its hood. Bend the spine backwards. Let the lower part of the body from the navel downwards right up to the toes touch the ground. Breathe normally through the nose. Retain the breath till the head is raised and the spine bent nicely. Then again exhale. Then retain the breath while bringing the head down, and as soon as the head touches the ground, slowly inhale again. Repeat this process of raising the head and bringing it down half a dozen times or more.

This is another good exercise for the spine. The spine becomes flexible and elastic. Rigidity and fatigue of the back are removed. Hunch-back, back pain, lumbago and myalgia of the back are relieved. Bhujangasana increases the intra-abdominal pressure and removes constipation. It augments appetite by increasing bodily heat and destroys a host of other ailments. This pose is specially useful for ladies to tone the ovary and uterus. It is a powerful tonic. Absence of menstruation (amenorrhoea) painful menstruation (dysmenorrhoea), whites (leucorrhoea) and various other utero-ovarine diseases are removed.

### (7)  SALABHASANA
#### (THE LOCUST POSE)

*Salabha* means a locust in Sanskrit. When this pose is demonstrated, it gives one the appearance of a locust.

Lie on the blanket face down and the arms touching the ground. Let the palms face upwards with the fingers clenched. Inhale slightly. Then stiffen the whole body and raise the legs, the hips and the lower abdomen up, putting the whole weight of the body on the chest and the hands. Raise the head also slightly.[13] Remain in this pose for 10 seconds in the beginning and prolong the time little by little as long as you can retain the breath. Bring the legs down slowly, relax the muscles of the whole body and exhale. Repeat this pose four or five times, taking care to see that the lungs are not unduly strained.

---

13.*Some specialists in Hatha-Yoga recommend the resting of the chin, mouth and nose on the ground, whilst some others the chin alone.*

This posture bends the spine backwards and gives intra-abdominal pressure. While Bhujangasana exercises the upper part of the body, Salabhasana develops the lower half of the body. It relieves constipation and tones the liver, pancreas and the kidneys. Several other diseases of the stomach are also removed. It is highly beneficial to persons suffering from lumbago. It increases the digestive fire, removes dyspepsia and promotes good appetite. A high standard of vitality and strength is assured.

## (8) DHANURASANA
### (THE BOW POSE)

*Dhanus* means a bow in Sanskrit. This is called Dhanurasana because when the full pose is demonstrated, it resembles a bow with a string in it. The hands and the legs represent the string, whereas the trunk and the thighs take the place of the bow.

As you did in the previous two poses, lie on the blanket face down. Relax all the muscles of the body. Bend the legs slowly at the knee-joint until the hands catch hold of the ankles. Raise the head, chest and knees. Keep the arms and the forearms stiff and straight. Try to keep the knees close together. Now the whole body rests on the abdomen. A good convex arch is formed resembling a bow with a string. You can either breathe as usual or retain the breath according to your convenience. Remain in this pose as long as you can comfortably do so. Do this Asana four to six times. When you have done this, lower the knees and the chest first. Then bring the hands and legs down and stretch flat on the ground.

This Asana gives the full benefits of both Bhujangasana and Salabhasana. The abdominal region gets a good massage. By rocking and swinging the bow-shaped body from side to side, forward and backward. a thorough massage and exercise to the abdomen is ensured. Chronic constipation, dyspepsia, sluggishness of the liver, rheumatism of the legs, knee-joints and the hands, gastro-intestinal disorders are all prevented and cured. Ladies desirous of undergoing a course of slimming will do well to try this Asana first. Dhanurasana keeps the spine strong and elastic. You will bubble with untiring energy, vigour and vitality. Everlasting youth is yours.

## (9) PASCHIMOTTANASANA
### (THE ANTERIOR SPINAL BENDING POSE)

Lie flat on the blanket and stretch the arms over the head. Slowly breathe in. Raise the arms, head and trunk, exhale and bend them over the legs, stretched taut, without raising the knees. Catch hold of the toes with the fingers, contracting the abdomen and gently pressing the head against the knees. Pull the toes with the arms and lower the elbows. While bending the trunk down, do not make any violent jerk. Do it very, very carefully and slowly. While remaining in this pose breathe normally. Remain in this pose for 2 seconds to start with and gradually increase the time to 10 minutes.

Paschimottanasana tones up the thigh and hamstring muscles. This is another excellent exercise for slimming purposes. This is a rare specific for obesity. Constipation is relieved. Sluggishness of the liver, dyspepsia, belching and gastritis are removed. Lumbago is cured. This is prescribed for piles and diabetes also. He who practises this posture regularly need not be afraid of old age. To him belongs eternal youth.

## (10) MAYURASANA
### (THE PEACOCK POSE)

*Mayura* means a peacock in Sanskrit. This is called Mayurasana because when this Asana is performed, it imitates a peacock spreading out his bundle of feathers behind him.

Kneel on the ground and squat on the heels. Bring the two forearms together and keep the palms on the ground. The palms and fingers represent the feet and claws of the peacock, except that here the palms are directed backward. Keep the elbowjoints in close contact with each other so as to provide a nice fulcrum to support the horizontal body during the display of the posture. The joint elbows are placed on the abdomen just below the navel. Stretch the whole body from head to foot up; so that it stands running parallel to the ground. Now the whole body looks like a bar resting on a fulcrum. Raise the head up and throw out the chin to counter-balance the heavy legs.

In the beginning retain the breath as long as you stand on this pose. Keep a thick and soft pillow or cushion on the ground just below your nose so as to protect in case of any slip. When you become perfect in this pose and there is no fear of falling down, you can breathe as usual during the exercise also. Beginners may practise the posture by balancing the body at the side of a table or a raised dais. It will be easy. Do this for 3 seconds to begin with and gradually prolong the time for 3 minutes.

Mayurasana promotes digestion and increases appetite. It is very potent in cases of dyspepsia and chronic gastritis. The bowels are toned up, and constipation is cured. All diseases of the stomach, liver, spleen, kidneys and the intestines are dispelled. Diabetes, haemorrhoids and piles are removed. The arms and shoulders become strong and sinewy.

## (11) BANDHA TRAYA
### (THE THREE BANDHAS)

That posture or exercise which shuts the gate of the body at a particular place and thereby stops inhalation and exhalation is called a Bandha. When Mula Bandha, Jalandhara Bandha and Uddiyana Bandha are practised at one and the same time, there ensues Bandha Traya.

Sit on Siddhasana pressing the perineum with the left heel and the other heel on the root of the generative organ. Inhale deeply. Contract the anus and draw it upwards. This is Mula Bandha. While in this state, contract the throat and press the chin tightly against the chest. This is Jalandhara Bandha. Then emptying the lungs by a complete exhalation, contract and draw up the intestines above and below the navel towards the spinal column. Now the abdomen rests against the back of the body high up in the thoracic cavity. This is called Uddiyana Bandha.[14]

---

14 *Uddiyana Bandha can also be done separately without mixing it with any other exercise. Though only the sitting posture is shown in the illustration, Uddiyana Bandha can be done in standing posture and various other postures as well.*

The practice of Bandha Traya is extremely helpful in establishing yourself in Brahmacharya. It gives vigour to the nerves, relieves constipation, and augments appetite. Blooming health, vigorous strength and a high standard of vitality are yours by right. The abdominal muscles are massaged and toned up. Persons suffering from chronic diseases of the stomach and the intestines and having given up all hopes of recovery will do well to try this natural remedy as a last resort. Rapid and marvellous cure is assured. Bandha Traya can be practised during Pranayama, concentration and meditation with much advantage. The Kundalini-Shakti is awakened and all psychic powers are bestowed upon the practitioner. He drinks the nectar of immortality and gets final emancipation (Moksha) .

### (12)  NAULI

*(ISOLATION OF THE RECTUS ABDOMINIS)*

The contraction, isolation and the rolling manipulation of the rectus abdominis is termed Nauli.

Stand up. Keep the legs a foot or so wide apart. Press your hands against the thighs by slightly bending the trunk. Then do Uddiyana Bandha in this standing posture. Let go the centre of the abdomen free by contracting the left and the right sides of the abdomen. Now all the muscles of the abdomen stand out bulging in the centre forming a vertical line. This is Nauli.[15] Remain in this pose as long as you can conveniently do so.

---

15 *The isolation of the abdominal muscles in the centre is called Madhyama Nauli. The isolation of the abdominal muscles on the left side is calleld Vamana Nauli and on the right side Dakshina Nauli.*

Constipation, dyspepsia and gastro-intestinal disorders are all thoroughly eradicated. The liver and the pancreas, the stomach and the intestines are toned up nicely. The muscles of the back and the intestines are strengthened and regenerated. Nauli is a rare gift to humanity right from the land of the gods and is an ideal 'pick-me-up.'

## Lesson VII

# PRANAYAMA

**P**rana means *breath* and *Ayama* means *control.* By Pranayama is meant the control of Prana and the vital forces of the body. Pranayama begins with the regulation of breath and ends in establishing full and perfect control over the life-currents or inner vital forces. In other words, Pranayama is the perfect control of the life-currents through regulation of breath. Breath like electricity is gross Prana. By establishing control over the gross Prana, you can easily gain control over the subtle Prana inside. The process by which such control is established is called Pranayama. Pranayama is the fourth limb of Ashtanga Yoga.

Prana is the oldest for, it starts functioning from the very moment the child is conceived. On the contrary, the organs of the body such as hearing, and so forth, begin to function only when their special abodes viz., the ears, etc., are formed. Prana is called the oldest and the best in the Upanishads because it gained the victory in the fight between mind and the five organs. In the end mind and the five organs unanimously declared: "O Master! O Prana! the supporter of this universe and the supporter of our very lives, the first-born! Adorations unto thee! Thou art really great. Do not depart from this body. We shall serve thee.

We duly acknowledge thy superiority." Prana functions even while the mind is absent during deep sleep.

Prana is the link between the physical and the astral bodies. When the slender thread-like Prana is cut off, the astral body separates from the physical body. Death is the result. The Prana that was working in the physical body is withdrawn into the astral body.

The sum total of the Rajasic portion of the five subtle elements forms the Pranas which are five in number,[16] and separately forms the hands and the other four organs of action. The five organs of action are contained in the Pranamaya Kosha (vital air sheath).

Prana digests the food, turns it into chyle and blood and sends it into the brain and mind. The mind is then able to think and do reflection (meditation) on the Self.

Prana is the universal principle of energy or force. It is vital force. Prana is all-pervading. It may be either in a static or dynamic state. It is found in all forms, from the lowest to the highest, from the ant to the elephant, from the unicellular amoeba to a man, from the elementary form of plant life to the developed form of animal life. It is Prana that shines in your eyes. It is through the power of Prana that the ear hears, the eye sees, the skin feels, the tongue tastes, the nose smells, the brain and the intellect perform their respective functions. The smile on the face of a young

---

16The five Pranas are: 1. Prana, 2. Apana, 3. Samana, 4. Vyana and 5. Udana.

lady, the melody in music, the power in the emphatic utterances of an orator, the charm in the words of one's own beloved wife—all these and many more have their origin in Prana. Fire burns through Prana. Wind blows through Prana. Rivers flow through Prana. The steamer and the aeroplane, the train and the motor-car move about only through the power of Prana. Radio-waves travel through Prana. Prana is electron. Prana is proton. Prana is force. Prana is magnetism. Prana is electricity. It is Prana that pumps blood from the heart into the arteries. It is Prana again that does digestion, excretion and secretion.

Prana is expended by thinking, willing, acting, moving, talking, writing and so on. A strong and healthy man has an abundance of Prana or nerve-force or vitality. The Prana is supplied by food, water, air, solar energy, etc. The supply of Prana is received by the nervous system. The Prana is absorbed in breathing. The excess of Prana is stored up in the brain and nerve-centres. When the seminal energy is sublimated, it supplies abundance of Prana to the system.

A Yogi stores up enough and more of Prana by regular practice of Pranayama just as the storage battery stores up electricity. That Yogi who has in his store an amazingly large supply of Prana radiates strength and vitality all around. He is a big power-house. Those who come in contact with him imbibe Prana from him, and get strength, vigour, vitality and exhilaration of spirits. Just as oil flows from one vessel to another, Prana also actually flows steadily from a developed Yogi towards weak persons. This can be seen actually by the Yogi who has developed his inner Yogic vision.

If you can control Prana, you can control all the forces of the universe, physical and mental. A Yogi can also control the Omnipresent Manifesting Power from which all energies like magnetism, electricity, gravitation, cohesion, nerve-currents, vital forces or thought-vibrations and, in fact, the total forces of the universe take their origin.

If you can control the breath or Prana, the mind is also easily controlled. He who has controlled his mind has also controlled his breath. If the one is suspended, the other also gets suspended. If the mind and the Prana are both controlled, you get liberation from the round of births and deaths and attain Immortality.

There is intimate connection between mind, Prana and semen. If you can control your seminal energy, you can also control your mind and Prana.

Owing to the vibration of Prana the ten senses (the five organs of action and the five organs of knowledge) do their respective functions. If the Prana is controlled, all the senses come under your control. Go through the parables in the Kaushitaki and the Chhandogya Upanishads. You will find that the senses recognised in the end the superiority of Prana. You can live without food and drink for days together, but you cannot live without air even for a few minutes. What to speak of Prana then!

As long as you speak, you cannot breathe; then you offer the breath in the speech. As long as you breath, so long you cannot speak; then you offer the speech in the breath. These are the two never-ending immortal oblations. When you want to hear a faint sound, the breath gets suspended for a while. The porter carrying heavy bags of rice or wheat at the wharf instinctively fills his lungs with air and practises unconscious retention of breath (Pranayama) till the bag is lifted on to his back. This retention of breath augments his strength and vitality. It immediately provides him with an abundance of energy. It induces great concentration of mind. When you cross a small rivulet by jumping over, when you practise long jump and high jump and various other exercises at the parallel bar and trapezium, you practise retention of breath instinctively.

If the breath is unsteady, the mind also is unsteady. If the breath is steady and calm, the mind is also steady and calm. A Yogi gets longevity of life by the practice of Pranayama. Therefore the practice of Pranayama is indispensable requisite. Just as it takes a long time, patience and perseverance to tame a lion, an elephant or a tiger, so also you will have to tame this Prana gradually. Then it will come under your perfect control.

Just as a goldsmith removes the impurities of gold by heating it in the blazing furnace and blowing the blow-pipe vigorously, so also the student of Yoga should remove the various impurities of his body and mind by blowing his lungs, i.e., by the practice of Pranayama. The fundamental aim of Pranayama is to unite the Prana and the Apana and to take the united Pranapana slowly upwards towards the crown of the head. The fruit of Pranayama is the awakening of the sleeping Kundalini-Shakti.

The room in which you practise Pranayama must not be damp and ill-ventilated. It must be dry and airy. The practice can be carried on by the side of a river or a lake, at the top or foot of a hill or a secluded part of a pleasant and beautiful garden, or at any place where the unconcentrated mind gets concentrated easily due to the exceptionally good spiritual vibrations. Whatever place you may finally select, take particular care to see that it is free from chill and strong draught, mosquitoes, bugs, ants and all other flies or crawling insects. If you wish to practise Pranayama in your own house, have a separate room under lock and key. Do not allow anybody into the room, no, not even your dearest and nearest friends and relatives. Let it be free from all other disturbing elements. There seated on your favourite Asana with the mind firmly fixed on Truth, perform Pranayama daily. Then the Chitta or the mind-stuff gets absorbed in the Sushumna.[17] The Prana becomes steady; it does not fluctuate. In India the banks of the Ganga, the Jumna and the Kaveri are extremely favourable for the practice of Pranayama, Rishikesh (Himalayas), Brindavan, Varanasi, Uttarakashi and Ayodhya are all very nice places for the purpose.

---

17.*Sushumna is the most important of the Nadis (nerve-currents). Situated at the back of the anus it extends to the crown of the head (Brahmarandhra) and is invisible and subtle. It runs along the centre of the spinal column with the Ida and Pingala Nadis running to its left and right. If you sit for meditation when the Prana moves in the Sushumna, you will have deep meditation. The Kundalini-Sakti lying dormant at the Muladhara Chakra, when roused by the practice of Pranayama, passess through the Sushumna Nadi to the crown of the head. This is the goal of life. This is perfection.*

The practice of Pranayama should be commenced in spring and autumn because success is assured. In the beginning you can have two sittings, morning and evening and as you advance in your practices, you can·have four: morning, midday, evening and midnight. Your diet should be light and moderate. In the early stages, food of milk and ghee is ordained; also food consisting of wheat, green pulse and red rice is said to favour the progress. Assuming your favourite Asana, practise regulation of breath first for the purification of the nerves (Nadis). Sri Sankaracharya, the greatest exponent of the Advaita philosophy, that India has ever produced says in his famous commentary to the Svetasvatara Upanishad: "The mind whose dross has been cleared away by Pranayama, becomes fixed in Brahman; therefore Pranayama is prescribed. First the nerves are to be purified, then comes the power to practise Pranayama. Closing the right nostril with the thumb, through the left nostril, fill in air according to capacity; then without any interval, throw the air out through the right nostril, closing the left one. Again inhaling through the right nostril, eject through the left, according to capacity; practising this three or five times at intervals of four hours of the day, before dawn, during midday, in the evening, and at midnight, in fifteen days or a month purity of the nerves is attained; then begins Pranayama." For complete success in Pranayama, regular persistent and systematic practice is essential.

Patanjali Maharshi defines Pranayama as follows: "Regulation of breath or the control of Prana is the stoppage of inhalation and exhalation, which follows after securing that steadiness of posture or seat." But you need not wait for practising Pranayama till you get full mastery over the posture. You can practise Asana and Pranayama side by side. In course of time you will acquire perfection in both. Pranayama can be practised while sitting in the chair also by sitting erect.

Each Pranayama cansists of three distinct processes viz., *Puraka* (inhalation of breath), *Kumbhaka* (retention of breath) and *Rechaka* (exhalation of breath). Kumbhaka gives longevity of life. If you can retain the breath for 10 seconds, know for certain that so many seconds have been added to the span of your life. By taking the breath to the crown of the head and keeping it there under his full and firm control, the Yogi defies and conquers death and drinks the Nectar of Immortality.

Pranayama is of three kinds according to the strength and capacity of the practitioner. The best one is that wherein Puraka is for 20 seconds,[18] Kumbhaka for 80 seconds and Rechaka for 40 seconds. The middling one is that wherein Puraka is for 16 seconds, Kumbhaka for 64 seconds and Rechaka for 32 seconds. The lowest one is that wherein Puraka is for 12 seconds, Kumbhaka for 48 seconds and Rechaka for 24 seconds. You should inhale and exhale very, very slowly, without producing any sound all the while. The ratio between Puraka, Kumbhaka and Rechaka is 1:4:2.

If there are impurities in the nerve-currents (Nadis), the Prana will not enter the middle Nadi, the Sushumna. In ordinary people the Sushumna is closed up at the lower end,

---

18Matra is the Sanskrit word for *second.* 1 Matra is equal to 1 second.

because of the various impurities of the body, mind and the nerves. When the nerves are purified, the Yogi can perform Pranayama with success. By the practice of Pranayama you can become a veritable god. Certain symptoms manifest when the Nadis are purified. Your body will become light and slender. There will be a peculiar lustre in your eyes and a remarkable glow in your countenance. Your voice will become sweet and melodious. The breath can be retained for a long time. You can hear the Anahata sounds emanating from your heart-lotus quite audibly. The digestive fire is augmented, you enjoy perfect health, and you are cheerful and happy.

The practice of concentration and Pranayama are interdependent. If you practise Pranayama, you will have concentration. Natural Pranayama follows the practice of concentration. A HathaYogi practises Pranayama and then controls the mind. He rises from a lower to a higher level; whereas a RajaYogi practises concentration and thus controls Prana. He comes down from a higher level. They both meet on a common platform in the end. There are different practices for different temperaments. For some the practice of Pranayama is easier to start with, for others the practice of concentration.

There is neither rhythm nor harmony in the breathing of worldly-minded persons. A Yogi practises regulation of breath to establish harmony. When the breath is regulated, when there is harmony, the breath will be moving within the nostrils. The fruit of regulation of breath is Kumbhaka. The breath stops by itself when Kevala Kumbhaka (absolute and pure retention of breath) follows. The mind becomes quite steady. Then Samadhi (superconscious state) supervenes. Regulation of breath and Kumbhaka are of tremendous help in the practice of concentration and meditation.

Dear child! Take sole refuge in Pranayama. Be interested in the practice of Kumbhaka alone, if the mind is solely turned towards Pranayama. The Bhagavad-Gita says: "*Pranayama-parayanah*—solely absorbed in the control of breathing." Take due precautions at every step. The practice of Kumbhaka produces tremendous heat in the body and thereby the Kundalini is roused and sent upwards along the Sushumna to the crown of the head.

Before I begin to deal with the various Pranayama exercises, I propose to give some preliminary instructions which would enable you to practise them without any difficulty and attain quick success in Yoga. The following are the most important:—

(1) All the instructions given in the last lesson hold good here also. You will have to use your common-sense and discretion throughout the practice of Yoga.

(2) The rule of celibacy will ensure quicker and better results. Those who cannot observe this rule very strictly for one reason or another, should be very, very moderate in copulation.

(3) Be regular and systematic in your practices.

(4) A small cup of milk or fruit-juice can be taken with much advantage before the commencement of the

practice, and another cup of milk and some light tiffin half an hour after the practice.

(5) *Do not miss your practice even a single day except when you are seriously ailing from some disease.*

(6) To start with, do mild Pranayama with Puraka and Rechaka only for a month. A rigid Pranayama-practitioner should abstain from all solid food. You can practise Pranayama while walking also. This will suit some busy persons who have not much time to spare.

(7) Practise the various exercises prescribed below one by one, step by step. Never be in a hurry. Never go beyond your capacity. Do not take up the higher exercise before completely mastering the previous one. This is the master-key to achieve success in Pranayama.

(8) There should be a feeling of joy and exhilaration after the Pranayama is over.

(9) Do not twist the facial muscles while doing Kumbhaka.

(10) Do not take bath for at least half an hour after the Pranayama exercises are over.

(11) Avoid as much as you can too much talking, eating, sleeping, mixing with friends and all exertion.

(12) Do not expect fruit after doing Pranayama for 2 or 3 minutes only for a few days. At least you must practise for 15 minutes daily in the beginning for some months.

(13) Success in Pranayama can be gauged by the duration of Kumbhaka. By slow and steady practice you will be able to retain the breath for at least 5 minutes. Real concentration of mind ensues when the breath is suspended.

(14) If you want rapid progress in Pranayama, you must have four sittings daily, at 4 a.m., at midday, at 4 p.m., and at midnight. You must do 4x80=320 Kumbhakas altogether.

(15) As there is always some drowsiness and laziness when you get up from bed, do a few Kumbhakas just to drive off the drowsiness and to make yourself fit for meditation.

In the first stage of Pranayama you will have perspiration of the body. You will experience a tremor of the body in the second stage. In the third stage levitation manifests. In the final stage the Prana goes to the Brahmarandhra (the Hole of Brahma) at the top of the head. Sometimes the practitioner may jump like a frog. When you perspire, do not use a towel to wipe off the perspiration. Rub it well on the body itself with your hands. This will give firmness and lightness to the constitution.

## EXERCISE

### I

(a) Sit on your favourite Asana before your Beloved Deity in your meditation room. Close the right nostril with the right thumb and slowly inhale through the left nostril as long as you can do with ease and comfort. Then exhale through the same nostril.[19]Do this half a dozen times. This will constitute one round. Do one round daily to begin with and gradually increase the number of rounds to 12.

(b) Inhale through the right nostril by closing the left nostril with the little and ring fingers of the right hand just in the same manner as you did before. Then exhale through the same nostril. Do this half a dozen times. This will constitute one round. Do one round daily to begin with and gradually increase the number of rounds to 12.

## II

Close the right nostril with the right thumb and inhale through the left nostril. Then close the left nostril with the little and ring fingers of the right hand and exhale through the right nostril after removing the thumb. Inhaling again through the right nostril and closing it with the thumb, exhale through the left nostril. Do in this manner half a dozen times. This will constitute one round. Do one round in the morning and one in the evening to begin with and gradually increase the number of rounds to 12 according to your capacity.

## III

Inhale through both the nostrils as much as you can and exhale through both the nostrils in the same manner.

---

19 *Feel that all the divine qualities such as love, mercy, forgiveness, peace, joy and knowledge enter your system along with the inspired air, and that all the devilish qualities such as lust, greed, anger and Avidya are thrown out along with the expired air. Also repeat mentally* OM *or* SOHAM *or any other Sacred Word given by your Guru during Puraka, Kumbhaka and Rechaka. This is the traditional method of doing Pranayama. This is the best method.*

Repeat this twelve times. This will constitute one round. Start with one round and increase the number of rounds gradually to six.

### IV

Draw the air in through both the nostrils as much as you can, retain it as long as you can, and then exhale as much as you can. Repeat this process twelve times. This will constitute one round. Start with one round and increase the number of rounds to six gradually.

### V

Close the right nostril with the right thumb and inhale through the left nostril. Then close the left nostril with the ring and little fingers of the right hand, retain the breath as long as you can comfortably do, and exhale through the right nostril by removing the thumb. Now half the process is over. Drawing again the air through the right nostril, and retaining it as before, exhale it through the left nostril by removing the ring and little fingers. These six processes constitute one Pranayama. Do 20 such Pranayamas in the morning and 20 in the evening to start with and gradually increase the number to 80.

If you wish to have time-unit, inhale till you count 1 OM; retain the breath till you count 4 OMs and exhale till you count 2 OMs. Observe the ratio 1:4:2. You may either use the left hand fingers for counting or mentally remember the numbers. In the second week increase the ratio to 2:8:4; in the third to 3:12:6, and so on and so forth until you reach the maximum of 20:80:40. While increasing the ratio, if you find it hard to retain the breath, have the same practice for two or three weeks more until the capacity and strength to increase the ratio further are gained. *Let there be no suffocation during the practice.*

## VI

Close the right ear with the right thumb, and the left ear with the left thumb. Press the right eye with the right index finger and the left eye with the left index finger. Place the middle finger of the right hand on the right nostril, and the middle finger of the other hand on the left. Let the ring fingers of the two hands press upon the upper lip, and the two tiny fingers upon the lower lip. Now inhale through both the nostrils as much as you can do with comfort; immediately close both the nostrils, and swallow the breath. Retain the breath inside as long as you can do with comfort and exhale it slowly. This is Shanmukhi Mudra. "The Yogi, by having thus firmly confined the air, sees his soul in the shape of light. When one sees, without obstruction this light even for a moment, becoming free from sin, he reaches the highest end. The Yogi, free from sin, and practising this continually, forgets his physical, subtle and causal bodies, and becomes one with that Soul. He who practises this in secrecy, is absorbed in the Brahman, though he had been engaged in sinful works. This should be kept secret; it at once produces conviction; it gives *Nirvana* to mankind. This is my most beloved Yoga." (Siva Samhita: Ch. V-22, 23, 24, 25, 26).

## VII

### RHYTHMICAL BREATHING

The breathing of worldly people is irregular. In exhalation the breath goes out 16 digits, and in inhalation only 12 digits, thus losing 4 clear digits of breath in every act of inspiration and expiration. Now just imagine how much Prana is wasted every day by you at this rate! If you can inhale 16 digits of Prana as in exhalation, everything is all right. There is absolutely no loss then. You will have rhythmical breathing. The Kundalini will be roused. Moreover, by practising this exercise and making it part and parcel of your daily life, you will enjoy perfect rest, a rest that you have never known or enjoyed even in your deep sleep.

The one striking feature of rhythmical breathing is that the time-unit is the same both in inhalation and exhalation. This is done in the following manner: Inhale till you mentally count 6 OMs and exhale till you count mentally 6 OMs. This is breathing in and out in a measured and harmonious manner. This kind of breathing will harmonise the whole system.

There is another variety in rhythmical breathing. You inhale through both the nostrils till you mentally count 4 OMs, retain the breath till you count 8 OMs and exhale through both the nostrils till you count 4 OMs. Then retain the breath outside (external Kumbhaka) till you count 8 OMs. These four processes constitute one Pranayama.

Do this as many times as your strength and capacity would allow. Gradually increase the duration of inhalation and exhalation till you count 16 OMs. There is no hurry. Enjoy every breath you inhale and exhale. Enjoy also the retention of breath. Pay good attention to the rhythm throughout. Feel the rhythm throughout your system. By slow and gradual practice with zeal and enthusiasm, you will attain perfection. Weep not! Grieve not! You are nearing the goal now, my child!

## VIII

## KAPALABHATI

Kapala means *a skull* and *Bhati* means to *shine*. Because this exercise makes your skull shine, it is called Kapalabhati. It is a wonderful exercise to cleanse the skull nicely. This exercise also does not come under the category of Pranayama, but as it is a breathing exercise, it deserves a place of honour.

Sitting on your usual meditative-pose, do Puraka and Rechaka so vigorously that you perspire profusely. There is no Kumbhaka in this exercise. But Rechaka plays a prominent part. Puraka is mild, slow and long and is best done by releasing the abdominal muscles, while Rechaka is forceful and quick and is done by contracting the abdominal muscle with a backward push. The important point to remember while doing this exercise is to keep the body, head and neck erect, and not to bend even a bit. In the beginning you can have one round only consisting of 10 expulsions in the morning. That will suffice. In the second week you can do the same in the evening also. In the third week have two rounds in the morning and two in the evening. In this manner you can cautiously and slowly increase 10 expulsions to each round till you get 120 expulsions per round.

The benefits of this exercise are even more alluring. The respiratory system and the nasal passages are thoroughly cleansed, the spasm in the bronchial tubes is removed, asthma is cured, the apices of the lungs are nicely oxygenized, consumption is cured and the impurities of the blood are eliminated. The circulatory and the respiratory systems are toned up beautifully, and the practitioner enjoys blooming health and vigour.

## IX

### SURYABHEDA

Sitting on your favourite meditative pose again and closing the eyes, inhale through the right nostril, retain the breath by forming Jalandhara Bandha till perspiration flows from the tips of the nails and the hairs of the body stand on end, and then exhale through the left nostril slowly. Of course in this exercise you cannot reach the point of perspiration at the very outset; but gradually increasing the period of Kumbhaka you will by all means attain it. By the constant practice of this Kumbhaka, cephalalgia is relieved, coryza is cured, and the worms in the frontal sinuses are expelled.

## X

### UJJAYI

The practice of this Kumbhaka enhances the personal beauty of the practitioner. Assuming again your favourite pose, inhale through both the nostrils in a smooth, methodical and uniform manner till the inspired breath fills the space between the throat and the stomach with a noise. Retain the breath as long as you can comfortably do and then exhale slowly through the left nostril. The striking feature of this exercise is that a mild, uniform, continuous and peculiar sound is heard due to the partial closure of the glottis.

This Kumbhaka is also practised while standing or walking. Then instead of exhaling through the left nostril only, you can exhale through both the nostrils. In any case, start with three rounds and add one round every week gradually.

The practitioner of this Kumbhaka gets rid of pulmonary, cardiac and dropsical diseases. All diseases dependent upon deficient inhalation of oxygen are cured.

## XI

### SITKARI

Folding the tongue in such a manner that the tip of the tongue touches the upper palate, draw the air through the mouth producing a sound of c. c. c., retain the breath as long as you can without the feeling of suffocation and then exhale through both the nostrils. These three processes constitute one round. Start with three rounds and add one round every week.

This Kumbhaka increases the beauty and vigour of the body, removes hunger and thirst, indolence and sleep and makes the whole body cool. Many diseases of the blood are cured.

## XII

### SITALI

Contract the lips and throw out the tongue. Fold the tongue like a tube and draw in the air through it making a hissing sound. Fill the lungs and stomach slowly with the air drawn in, and retain the same as long as you can do with comfort. Then exhale through both the nostrils. Practise this 10 to 20 times daily, morning and evening.

The practitioner acquires great tenacity of life and the power to repair the effects of injury. He is freed from all fevers, splenitis, and several other organic diseases. Like crabs, lobsters, serpents and frogs, he becomes proof against all kinds of inflammations. He acquires the power to cast off his skin and endure the privation of air, food and drink. Poisons of all sorts in the blood are thrown out and the blood is purified. Scorpion-stings and serpent-bites cannot injure him in any way. Whenever you feel thirsty, do this Pranayama a few times. At once your thirst will be quenched.

## XIII

### BHASTRIKA

*Bhastrika* means *bellows*. Quick succession of powerful expulsions of breath is the chief characteristic of this Pranayama. Just as the village smith blows out his bellows quickly and rapidly, so also the practitioner of this exercise blows out the bellows of his lungs in quick and rapid succession.

Sit on Padmasana or Siddhasana with the body, neck and head erect. Close the mouth. Inhale and exhale quickly 6 to 10 times in rapid succession like the bellows of the village-smith. While practising this Pranayama a hissing sound is loudly heard. If you can expel 10 times like this, the tenth expulsion is followed by a deepest inhalation, retained as long as it can be done with comfort, and another deepest exhalation. This completes one round of Bhastrika. Take rest for a while after one round is over, and do another round, and another round. In the beginning you can have three rounds in the morning and three in the evening. You must be able to expel 120 times at a stretch by cautious and gradual practice.

If you can do Kapalabhati and Ujjayi nicely, you will find this Pranayama quite easy. Some do this exercise till they get quite fatigued. Then you will profusely perspire. *Stop the practice even if there is the slightest giddiness. Take a few normal breaths.* Then you can resume the practice again after the giddiness is gone.

## XIV

### PLAVINI

This Pranayama requires some skill on the part of the practitioner. If you can do this perfectly, you can float on water for any length of time, even though you do not know swimming. It enables you to live purely on air for some days. It is done as follows: Drink the air like water through the mouth and fill your stomach with it. The stomach becomes inflated. You will hear a tympanic sound, if you tap it with your fingers. Practise the Pranayama slowly and gradually. The air is then expelled from the stomach by slow belching.

## XV

### KEVALA KUMBHAKA

Kumbhaka is of two sorts—*Sahita* and *Kevala*. The Kumbhaka that is associated with Puraka and Rechaka is called Sahita; that which is devoid of these two is called Kevala (pure and absolute). Kevala Kumbhaka should be practised when the Sahita Kumbhaka has been completely mastered. In the Vasishtha Samhita you will find: "When after giving up inhalation and exhalation, one holds his breath with ease, it is absolute Kumbhaka (Kevala Kumbhaka)." In this Pranayama the practitioner can retain his breath as long as he likes. He attains the stage of

Raja-Yoga. Practise this three times a day, morning, midday and evening. He is a real Yogi who knows this Kumbhaka and Pranayama. Now there is nothing unattainable by him in all the three worlds. This Kumbhaka cures all diseases, bestows longevity of life and awakens the Kundalini-Sakti, which passes through the hollow Sushumna-Nadi to the crown of the head, after piercing one Chakra after another.

## BENEFITS OF PRANAYAMA

Perfection in Pranayama gives you the major eight Siddhis viz., *Anima, Mahima, Laghima, Garima, Prapti, Prakamya, Vasitvam* and *Isitvam*. Anima is the power to become as minute as you like, whereas Mahima makes you as big as you like. By Laghima you can make your body as light as a feather and fly in the sky thousands of miles in a minute. Garima can make your body as heavy as a mountain. By the power of Prapti you can predict all future events, understand unknown languages, cure any disease, hear distant sounds, see distant objects, smell mystical fragrant odours, touch the sun and the moon with the tip of your fingers from where you stand, and understand the language of birds and beasts. Indeed you can attain all desired objects. By Prakamya you can cast away the old skin and assume a youth-like appearance for an unusual length of time. You can also enter the body of another person. Sri Sankaracharya had this power. He entered the body of the Raja of Benares. Yayati, Tirumulanar and Raja Vikramaditya had also this power. Vasitvam is the power to tame wild beasts and bring them under your control. By the exercise of this power, you can make anybody obey your orders and wishes. You can control the elements and be a master of passions and emotions. Isitvam is the attainment of all divine powers. You now become the Lord of the universe. You can give life to a dead man. Kabirdas, Tulasidas, Akalkot Swami and many others had this power. By possessing this power you can penetrate all secrets of nature, know the events of the past, present and future and become one with the Supreme Soul.

You will also get the thirty-six other minor Siddhis such as freedom from hunger and thirst, heat and cold, pleasure and pain; death at your will, playing with gods, power to transmute baser metals into gold and so on.[20]

---

20 *For further details refer to my book "Science of Pranayama."*

*Lesson VIII*

# CONCENTRATION

Hari Om! My speech is rooted in my mind,
My mind is rooted in my speech;
Brahman, reveal Thyself to me;
Ye mind and speech enable me
To grasp the truth the scriptures teach.
Let what I have heard slip not from me;
I join day with night in study,
I think the truth, I speak the truth;
May That protect me,
May That protect the teacher,
Protect me, protect the teacher, protect the teacher.
Om Peace! Om Peace! Om Peace!

*Desa-bandhas-chittasya dharana*—Concentration is fixing the mind on an external object or an internal point. Once a Sanskrit scholar approached Kabir[21] and asked him: "O Kabir! What are you doing now?" Kabir replied: "O Pandit! I am detaching the mind from worldly objects and attaching it to the Lotus Feet of the Lord." This is concentration. Right conduct, posture, Pranayama and abstraction from sensual objects will pave a long way in achieving rapid success in concentration. There can be no

---

21 *Kabir, a weaver saint of the holy city of Kasi, is said to have lived during the reign of Sikandar Lodhi and died in the year 1519 A.D. He was a distinguished disciple of the great religious reformer, Ramananda, and had marvellous psychic powers.*

concentration without something upon which the mind may rest. Concentration is the sixth step in the Yogic ladder.

You must evince good interest in the practice of concentration. Then only your whole attention will be directed towards the object upon which you wish to concentrate. There can be really no concentration without a remarkable degree of *interest* and *attention* shown by the practitioner. You must therefore, know what these two words mean.

Attention is steady application of the mind. It is focussing of consciousness on some chosen object. Through attention you can develop your mental faculties and capacities. Where there is attention, there is also concentration. Attention should be cultivated gradually. It is not a special process. It is the whole mental process in one of its aspects.

Perception always involves attention. To perceive is to attend. Through attention you get a clear and distinct knowledge of objects. The entire energy is focussed on the object towards which attention is directed. Full and complete information is gained. During attention all the dissipated rays of the mind are collected. There is effort or struggle in attention. Through attention a deeper impression of anything is made in the mind. If you have good attention, you can attend to the matter in hand exclusively. An attentive man has very good memory. He is very vigilant and circumspect. He is nimble and alert.

If you analyse carefully the mental functions or operations, no one process can be singled out and called attention to. It is not possible to separate attention as a distinct function. You observe something; therefore you are attentive.

Attention belongs to every state of consciousness and is present in every field of consciousness. An attentive student in the spiritual path can do hearing (Sravana) of the Srutis[22] in an efficient manner. The military officer says: "ATTENTION' and the soldier is ready with his gun to carry out his behests. An attentive soldier alone can hit the mark. No one can get success either in temporal or spiritual pursuits without attention.

There are Yogins who can do eight or ten or even hundred things at a time[23]. This is not strange. The whole secret lies in the fact that they have developed their attention to a remarkable degree. All the great men of the world do possess this faculty in varying degrees.

Attention is of two kinds viz., external attention and internal attention. When the attention is directed towards external objects, it is called external attention. When it is directed internally within the mind upon mental objects and ideas, it is known as internal attention.

There are again two other kinds of attention viz, voluntary attention and involuntary attention. When the attention is directed towards some external object by an effort, of the will, it is called voluntary attention. When

---

22*Hindu Scriptures such as the Upanishads Brahma-Sutras, etc.*

23Read my book "*Mind, Its Mysteries and Control.*"

you have an express volition to attend to this or that, it is called involuntary attention. The man understands why he perceives. Some deliberate intention, incentive, goal or purpose is definitely involved. Voluntary attention needs effort, will, determination and some mental training. This is cultivated by practice and perseverance. The benefits derived by the practice of attention are incalculable. Involuntary attention is quite common. This does not demand any practice. There is no effort of the will. The attention is induced by the beauty and attractive nature of the object. Individuals perceive without knowing why and without observed instruction. Young children possess this power of involuntary attention to a greater degree than grown-up people.

If a man is not observant, he is not attentive. If he observes something, he is said to be attentive. Intention, purpose, hope, expectation, desire, belief, wish, knowledge, aim, goal and needs serve to determine attention. You will have to note carefully the degree, duration, range, forms, fluctuations and conflicts of attention.

There is great attention, if the object is very pleasing. You will have to create interest. Then there will be attention. If the attention gets diminished, change your attention to another pleasant object. By patient training you can direct the mind to attend to an unpleasant object also by creating interest. Then your will will grow strong.

If you closely watch, you will note that you observe different objects at different times. This perception of now one object and now another when the physical conditions are constant, is known as fluctuation of attention. Attention is changing. The objects themselves change or fluctuate but there is no fluctuation in the observing individual himself. The mind has not been trained to bear prolonged voluntary attention. It gets disgusted through monotony and wants to run towards some other pleasing object. You may say: "I am going to attend to one thing only," but you will soon find that even though you attend very hard, you suddenly perceive something else. The attention wavers.

Interest develops attention. It is difficult to fix the mind on an uninteresting object. When a professor is lecturing, when the subject is abstract and metaphysical, many people leave the hall quietly because they cannot attend to a subject which is not interesting. But if the same professor sings and tells some interesting and thrilling stories, all people hear him with rapt attention. There is pindrop silence. Lecturers should know the art of attracting the minds of the hearers. They will have to change the tone to talk with force and emphasis. They will have to watch the audience and see whether they are attentive or not. They will have to change the subject-matter for a short while and bring in some nice stories and suitable illustrations. They will have to look at the hearers directly in their eyes. So many things are necessary if one wants to become a successful lecturer, if one wants to make the hearers attentive.

Napoleon, Gladstone, Arjuna and Jnanadeva had all wonderful powers of attention. They could fix their minds on any object. All scientists and occultists possess attention to a remarkable degree. They cultivate it by patience, regular and systematic practice. A judge and a surgeon can get positive success in their respective professions only if they are endowed with the power of attention to a high degree.

When you do any work, plunge yourself in it. Forget yourself. Lose the self. Concentrate upon the work. Shut out all other thoughts. When you do one thing, do not think of any other thing. When you study one book, do not think of any other book. Fix the mind there steadily like the arrow-maker[24] who had no consciousness of his surroundings. Eminent scientists are so busy and attentive in their experiments and researches in their laboratories that they forget to take food even for days together. Once a scientist was very busy at his work. His wife who was living in another district had a serious calamity. She came running up to him to the laboratory with profuse tears in her eyes. Strange to say, the scientist was not a bit agitated. He was so very attentive in his work that he even forgot that she was his own wife. He replied: "Madam! Weep for some more time. Let me make chemical analysis of your tears."

Once some gentleman invited Sir Isaac Newton for dinner. Newton repaired to his host's bungalow and took his seat in the drawing room. The gentleman forgot all about Newton, took his dinner and proceeded to his office. Newton was amusing within himself very absorbedly on some important point of science. He did not stir from his

---

24 *There was a workman who used to manufacture arrows. Once he was very busy at his work. He was so much engrossed in his work that he did not notice a Raja and his retinue passing in front of his work-shop. Such must be the nature of your concentration, when you fix your mind on God. You must have the one idea of God and God alone.*

seat. He forgot all about his dinner and remained in the same chair like a statue for over thirtysix hours! The next morning the host saw Newton in the drawing room and then only remembered of having invited him for dinner. He really felt sorry for his forgetfulness and apologised to Sir Isaac in a meek voice. What a wonderful power of attention Sir Isaac Newton had! All geniuses possess this power to an infinite degree.

According to Prof. James we attend to things because they are very interesting. But Prof. Pillsbury is of the opinion that things are interesting because we attend to them, or because we are likely to attend to them. We do not attend to them because they are interesting.

By the constant practice and ever-renewed effort of attention, a subject that in the beginning was dry and uninteresting may become full of interest when you master it and learn its meaning and its issues. The power of concentrating your attention on the subject may become stronger.

When a great misfortune has befallen you, or when you pass in review a certain course of conduct in order to find out the cause of failure, it may take possession of your mind to such a degree that no effort of the will can make you cease from thinking over it. An article has to be written, a book is in the process of preparation; the work is carried on to the loss of sleep and you are unable to tear yourself away from it; the attention which began voluntarily has taken entire hold of the field of consciousness.

If you possess strong power of attention, anything that the mind receives will be deeply impressed. An attentive man only can develop his will. A mixture of attention, application and interest can work wonders. There is no doubt of this. A man of ordinary intellect with highly developed attention can turn out more work than a highly intellectual man who has a poor attention. Failure in anything is mainly due to lack of attention. If you attend to one thing at a time, you will get profound knowledge of that subject in its various aspects. The ordinary untrained man of the world generally attends to several things at a time. He allows many things to enter the gates of his mental factory. That is the reason why he has a clouded or turbid mind. There is no clarity of thought. He cannot do the process of analysis and synthesis. He is bewildered. He cannot express his ideas clearly, whereas the disciplined man can attend to a subject exclusively as long as he likes. He extracts full and detailed information about one subject or object and then takes up another. Attention is an important faculty of a Yogi.

You cannot attend to two different objects at a time. Mind can do only one thing at a time. Because it moves with such tremendous velocity backwards and forwards, you think that the mind can attend to several objects or things at a time. You can only see or hear at a time. You cannot see and hear at the same time. But this law is not applicable to a developed Yogi. A developed Yogi can do several things at a time because his will is not separate from the Cosmic Will which is all-powerful. Psychology is only a product of the Cosmic Will, and as such it has not got the strength to dominate over it.

Before you begin the practice of concentration, you will do well to know something about the subconscious mind and its functions. In the Vedanta philosophy the subconscious mind is called *Chitta*. When the Chitta is confined and fixed to a certain point or object, this is called concentration. A great deal of your subconsciousness is but bundles of submerged experiences which can be brought to the surface of the conscious mind by means of concentration.

It is an admitted psychological fact that the mental processes by which you obtain knowledge are not merely confined to the field of consciousness but also cover the field of subconsciousness. If you know the technique of speaking to your subconscious mind and the art or science of extracting work from it just as you would speak to your servant or a dear old friend, then all knowledge will be yours. Yes, it is a question of practice, and practice will make you perfect.

When you are unable to solve some puzzle in metaphysics, science or philosophy, ask your subconscious mind to do the bit of work for you with the full trust and confidence that you are bound to get the right solution from it. Command your subconscious mind in the following manner: "Look here, you subconscious mind; I want the solution to this puzzle or problem very urgently tomorrow morning. Kindly do it quickly." Let your command be given in very clear terms, and let there be no ambiguity about it. You will positively get the answer from your subconscious mind the next morning. But sometimes the subconscious mind may be busy otherwise and in such cases you will have to wait for some days. You will have to repeat the command regularly every day at a fixed time.

All that you have inherited, all that you have brought with you through innumerable crores of births in the past, all that you have seen, heard, enjoyed, tasted, read or known either in this life or in past lives are hidden in your subconscious mind. Why don't you master the technique of concentration and the way of commanding your subconscious mind and make full and free use of all that knowledge?

The subconscious mind is, as you have already known, your faithful servant. When at night you retire to bed with the thought that you should get up positively at 4 a.m., to either catch a train or practise meditation, it is your subconscious mind that wakes you up at the exact hour. Even while you are fast asleep, your subconscious mind is at work. It has no rest at all. It arranges. analyses, compares, sorts all facts and figures, and finally carries out your commands.

Every action, every enjoyment or suffering and, in fact, all experiences leave in the camera-plate of your subconscious mind subtle impressions or residual potencies which are the root cause of future births, experiences of pleasure and pain, and death again. Revival or repetition of any action done in this life induces memory. But in the case of a developed Yogi memory of previous lives also is brought about. He dives deep within and comes in actual contact with the Samskaras (subtle impressions) of past lives. He directly perceives them through his Yogic Vision. By means of Yogic Samyama (concentration, meditation and Samadhi practised at one and the same time) the Yogi gets full knowledge of past lives. By doing Samyama on the Samskaras of others, he gets knowledge of the past lives of others also. Wonderful are the powers of concentration.

Mind is a power born of Atman because it is through mind that God manifests Himself as the differentiated universe of names and forms. Mind is nothing but a bundle of thoughts and habits. As the "I" thought is the root of all thoughts, mind is only the thought "I"

The brain is the seat of the mind in the waking state; the cerebellum in the dreaming state; and the heart in the deep sleep state. All objects you see about you, are nothing but mind only in form and in substance. Mind creates; mind destroys. A higher developed mind influences the lower minds. Telepathy, mind-reading, hypnotism, mesmerism, distant healing and so many other allied sciences bear testimony to the fact. Undoubtedly mind is the greatest power on earth. Control of mind bestows all powers.

Just as you take physical exercises, play games such as tennis and cricket in order to maintain physical health, you will have to maintain mental health also by taking Sattvic food, mental recreation of innocent and harmless nature, change of thought, relaxation of mind by entertaining good, ennobling and sublime thoughts and by cultivating the habit of cheerfulness.

The nature of the mind is such that it becomes that which it intensely thinks upon. Thus, if you think of the vices and defects of another man, your mind will be charged with those defects and vices at least for the time being. He who knows this psychological law will never indulge in censuring others or in finding fault in the conduct of others. He will always praise others. He will only see the good in others. That is the way to grow in concentration, Yoga and spirituality.

Mind is atomic according to the Indian school of logic; all-pervading according to the RajaYoga philosophy; and is of the same size as that of the body according to the Vedantic school.

Deep sleep is not a state of inactivity. In this state the causal body (Karana Sarira) functions vigorously. The associated consciousness, Prajna, is also present. The Jiva (individual soul) is almost in close contact with the Absolute. Just as a thin layer of muslin veils the face of a lady and renders it invisible to the eyes of her husband, so also, a thin layer of ignorance separates the individual soul and the Supreme Soul. Students of Vedanta study this state deeply. It has deep philosophical significance. It gives the clue to trace the existence of the Atman. You rest in the warm bosom of the Mother of the world, Rajesvari, who lovingly bestows upon you peace, refreshing vigour and strength to face the ensuing battle of daily life. But for this incomparable love and kindness of the merciful Mother during deep sleep, life would be well nigh impossible on this physical plane, where so many miseries, diseases, cares, worries, anxieties and fears of all sorts torture and torment you every moment. How miserable, gloomy and depressed you feel, if you do not enjoy sound sleep even for one night, if you happen to forgo your sleep for three or four hours by attending a night's theatrical entertainment!

Great Yogins like Jnanadeva, Bhartrihari and Patanjali used to send and receive messages to and from distant persons through mind-telepathy (mental radio) and thought-transference. Telepathy was the first wireless telegraph and telephone service ever known to the world. Thought travels with tremendous velocity through space. Thought moves. It has weight, shape, size, form and colour. It is a dynamic force.

What is this world after all? It is nothing but the materialisation of the thoughtforms of Hiranyagarbha or God. You have got waves of heat, and light and electricity in science. There are also thought-waves in Yoga. Thought has tremendous power. Everybody is experiencing the power of thought unconsciously to a greater or lesser degree. If you have a comprehensive understanding of the working of thought-vibrations, if you know the technique of controlling the thoughts, if you know the method of transmitting beneficial thoughts to others at a distance by forming clearcut, well-defined powerful thought-waves, you can use this thought-power a thousandfold more effectively. Thought works wonders. A wrong thought binds. A right thought liberates. Therefore think rightly and attain freedom.

Dear child! Unfold the occult powers hidden within you by understanding and realising the powers of the mind. Close your eyes. Slowly concentrate. You can see distant objects, hear distant sounds, send messages to any part of, not only, this world but to other planets as well, heal persons thousands of miles off from you, and move about to distant places in no time. Believe in the powers of the mind.

Interest, attention, will, faith and concentration will bring the desired fruit. Remember that mind is born of the Atman through His Maya (illusory Power).

Cosmic mind is universal mind. Cosmic mind is the sum total of all individual minds. Cosmic mind is Hiranyagarbha or Isvara or Karya Brahman. Man's mind is only a fragment of the universal mind. Learn to merge your little mind in the Cosmic mind and get Omniscience and experience Cosmic Consciousness.

Keep a balanced mind always. This is a very important thing. It is, no doubt, a difficult practice, but you will have to do it, if you wish to succeed in concentration. Keeping the balance of mind in pleasure and in pain, in heat and in cold, in gain and in loss, in success and in failure, in praise and in censure, in respect and in disrespect, is real wisdom. This is very trying indeed, but if you are able to do this, you are a mighty potentate on earth. You are fit to be adored. You are the most wealthy man, though you are clad in loin-cloth, though you have nothing to eat. You are very strong, though you have a dilapidated physical frame. Worldly people lose their balance even for trifling things. They get irritated and lose their temper quickly. Energy is wasted when one loses his temper. Those who want to develop balance of mind should develop discrimination and practise celibacy and concentration. Those who waste their semen get irritated very frequently. Control and concentration of mind is very difficult of performance, for, Saint Thayumanavar in his inimitable poem "Tejomayanandam" has written a beautiful verse on the

difficulty of controlling the mind.[25] This untranslatable
piece roughly and freely translated means:

"You can control a mad elephant;
You can shut the mouth of the bear and the tiger;
You can ride on a lion;
You can play with the cobra;
By alchemy you can eke out your livelihood;
You can wander through the universe incognito;
You can make vassals of the gods;
You can ever be youthful;
You can walk on water;
You can live in fire;
You can achieve all Siddhis, seated in your home;
But to be restful by control of the mind is rare
　　　　　　　　　　　　　　　　　and difficult."

The senses are your real foes. They draw you out and
perturb your peace of mind. Do not keep company with
them. Subdue them. Restrain them. Curb them just as you
would curb your enemies on the battlefield. This is not a
day's work. It demands patient and protracted Sadhana for a
very long time. Control of the senses is really control of the
mind. All the ten senses must be controlled. Starve them to
death. Do not give them what they want. Then they will
obey your orders quite implicitly. All worldly-minded
persons are slaves of their senses, though they are educated,
though they possess immense wealth, though they hold
judicial and executive powers. If you are a slave of

25 *Thayumanavar was a poet-saint who lived about 200 years ago in the
district of Tanjore, South India. His songs on Vedanta are
soul-inspiring and elevating. All his songs are now available in
gramophone records. They penetrate deep into the hearts of the
hearers. They are very, very popular in South Inida. They are pregnant
with deep, subtle, philosophical thoughts.*

meat-eating, for instance, you will begin to exercise control over·your tongue the moment you give up the meat-eating habit entirely for six months. You will consciously feel that you have gained a little supremacy over this troublesome sense of taste which began to revolt against you sometime ago.

Be cautious, vigilant and circumspect. Watch your mind and its modifications. Lord Jesus says: "Watch and pray". Watching the mind is introspection. One in a million does this beneficial and soul-elevating practice. People are immersed in worldliness. They madly run after money and women. They have no time to think of God and higher spiritual things. The sun dawns and the mind runs again in its old, usual, sensual grooves of eating, drinking, amusing and sleeping. The day has passed. In this way the whole life passes away. There is neither moral development nor spiritual progress. He who does daily introspection can find out his own defects and remove them by suitable methods and can have gradually a perfect control over the mind. He will not allow the intruders—lust, anger, greed, delusion and pride—to enter the mental factory. He can practise concentration uninterruptedly.

Daily self-analysis and self-examination is another indispensable practice. Then only you can obviate your defects and grow rapidly in concentration. What does a gardener do? He watches the young plants carefully, removes the weeds daily, puts a strong fence round them and waters them daily at the proper time; and so they grow nicely and yield fruits quickly. Even so you should find out your defects by introspection and self-analysis and eradicate them through suitable methods. If one method fails, you should take recourse to another. The practice demands patience, perseverance, leech-like tenacity, application, iron will, subtle intellect and courage. But the reward is invaluable. It is Immortality, Supreme Peace and Infinite Bliss!

You should try to possess a serene mind. You should practise serenity every moment of your Yogic career. If your mind is restless, you cannot make an iota of progress in concentration. Therefore, the first and foremost thing that you should possess by all means is serenity of mind. Silent meditation in the morning, renunciation of desires, suitable diet, discipline of the senses and observance of the vow of silence daily for about at least an hour will produce serenity. All vain, habitual thoughts, wild fancies, wrong feelings, cares, worries, anxieties, confused ideas, and all kinds of imaginary fears must be done away with in toto. Then and then only you can hope to get a peaceful mind. The foundation in Yoga can well and truly be laid only if the aspirant possesses serenity to a maximum degree. Only a calm mind can grasp the truth, can see God or Atman, can receive the Divine Light. The spiritual experiences will be permanent, if you have a quiet mind. Otherwise they will come and go.

As soon as you wake up in the morning, pray fervently to the Lord, sing His Names, and meditate upon Him with all your heart from 4 to 6. Then make a firm determination: "I will observe celibacy today. I will speak the truth today. I will not hurt the feelings of others today. I will not lose my temper today." Watch your mind. Be resolute. You will surely succeed that day. Then continue the vow for the whole week. You will gain strength. Your will-power will develop. Then continue the vow for the whole month. Even if you commit some mistakes in the beginning; you need not be unnecessarily alarmed. Mistakes are your best teachers. You will not commit the same mistakes again. If you are earnest and sincere, the Lord will shower His Grace upon you. The Lord will give you strength to face the difficulties and troubles in the daily battle of life.

He who has controlled his mind is really happy and free. Physical freedom is no freedom at all. If you are easily carried away by surging emotions and impulses, if you are under the grip of moods, cravings and passions, how can you be really happy, O sweet beloved child! You are like a rudderless boat. You are tossed about hither and thither like a piece of straw in the vast expanse of the ocean. You laugh for five minutes and weep for five hours. What can wife, son, friends, money, fame and power do for you, when you are under the sway of the impulses of your mind? He is the true hero who has controlled his mind. There is an adage: "He who has controlled his mind has controlled the world." True victory is over the mind. That is real freedom. Thorough rigorous discipline and self-imposed restrictions will eventually eradicate all desires, thoughts, impulses, cravings and passions. Only then and not until then can you expect to be free from the thraldom of the mind. You should not give any leniency to the mind. The mind is a mischievous imp. Curb it by drastic measures. Become a perfect Yogi. Money cannot give you freedom. Freedom is not a commodity that can be purchased in the Crawford Market. It is a rare hidden treasure guarded by a five-hooded serpent. Unless you kill or tame this serpent, you cannot have access to this treasure. That treasure is Spiritual Wealth, that is Freedom, that is Bliss. The serpent is your mind. The five-hoods are the five senses through which the mind-serpent hisses.

Rajasic mind always wants new things. It wants variety. It gets disgusted with monotony. It wants change of place, change of food, change, in short, of everything. But you should train the mind to stick to one thing. You should not complain of monotony. You should have patience, adamantine will and untiring persistence. Then only you can succeed in Yoga. He who wants something new always is quite unfit for Yoga. You should stick to one place, one spiritual preceptor, one method and one system of Yoga. That is the way to positive success.

You should have real and intense thirst for God-realisation. Then all obstacles will be obviated. Concentration will be quite easy for you then. Mere emotional bubbling for the time being out of sheer curiosity or for attaining psychic powers cannot bring any tangible result.

If you are careless, if you are irregular in concentration, if your dispassion (Vairagya) wanes, if you give up the practice for some days on account of laziness, the adverse forces will take you away from the true path of Yoga. You will be stranded. It will be difficult for you to rise up again to the original height. Therefore be regular in concentration.

Be cheerful and happy. Away with depression and gloom. There is nothing more infectious than depression. A depressed and gloomy man can radiate only unpleasant and morbid vibrations all around; he cannot radiate joy, peace and love. Therefore never come out of your room, if you are depressed and gloomy lest you should spread the contagion all around you. Live only to be a blessing to others. Radiate joy, love and peace. Depression eats the very core of your being and havocs like a canker. It is verily a deadly plague. Depression manifests on account of some disappointment or failure, severe dyspepsia or heated debates, wrong thinking or wrong feeling. Separate yourself from this negative feeling and identify yourself with the Supreme Being. Then no external influence can affect you. You will be invulnerable. Drive the feeling of depression and gloom at once by enquiry, singing divine songs, prayers, chanting of OM, Pranayama, a brisk walk in the open air, thinking of the opposite quality viz., the feeling of joy. Try to be happy in all states and radiate joy only towards all around you.

Why do you weep, my child? Remove the bandage from your eyes and see now. You are surrounded by truth and truth alone. All is Light and Bliss only. The cataract of ignorance has blurred your vision. Extract the cataract immediately. Put on a new pair of glasses by developing the inner eye of wisdom through regular practice of concentration.

It is not thought alone that determines action. There are some intelligent people who think reasonably on the pros and cons of a thing but when the time comes they are led astray by temptations. They do wrong actions and repent later on. It is the feeling that really goads man to action. Some psychologists lay special stress on imagination and say that it is imagination that really determines action. They bring the following illustration in support of their view: Suppose a long plank 1 foot broad is placed between two turrets each 20 feet high. When you begin to walk on this plank, you imagine that you will fall down and so you actually fall down. Whereas you are able to walk on the same plank when placed on the ground. Suppose you go on a bicycle along a narrow lane. You see a big stone on the way. You imagine that you will hit the cycle against the stone; and so you actually run the cycle against the stone. Some other psychologists say that it is the will that determines an action. Will can do everything. Will is soul-force. Vedantins are of this latter opinion.

Now to come back to the subject of concentration proper: The waves in the mind caused by thought-forms are called *Vrittis*. These waves must be stilled or stopped. Then only you can realise the Soul. A well-trained mind can be fixed at will upon any object either inside or outside to the exclusion of all else. The practice of concentration is a bit disgusting in the beginning but it will give you immense happiness after sometime. Patience and perseverance are essential. Regularity is also necessary. The mind is compared in the Hindu Sastras to a lake or ocean. The thoughts arising from the mind are compared to the waves of the ocean. You can see your reflection clearly on the waters of the ocean only when all the waves on the surface subside completely and become still. So also you can realise the Soul, the Light of lights, only when all the thought-waves in the mind-lake are stilled.

If you take interest in the practice of concentration, and if you have a definite purpose, you will have remarkable progress in concentration. Some medical students leave the medical college soon after joining as they find it disgusting to wash the pus in ulcers and wounds and dissect dead bodies. Is it not a serious blunder? In the beginning, no doubt, it is loathsome; but after studying pathology, medicine, operative surgery, morbid anatomy, bacteriology and so on, the course becomes very interesting in the final year. When they begin to get some knowledge of medicine, diagnosis and treatment, and when they begin to think of the prospects of earning much money after qualifying themselves as doctors, they begin to evince great interest in the line.

Many spiritual aspirants leave off the practice of concentration after sometime as they find it difficult to practise it. In this they commit a grave blunder like the medical students. In the beginning of the practice, when you struggle hard to get over body-consciousness, it will be disgusting and troublesome. But in the third year of the practice the mind will become cool, pure and strong. The neophyte will find great interest in the practice, when he gets some psychic experiences such as brilliant lights, hearing of celestial sounds, smelling of rare scents, and so on, and when he begins to think of the prospects of becoming a fully developed Yogi.

Some people can concentrate on pleasant or interesting objects only. If they can create interest in unpleasant things also, they can do good concentration on uninteresting things as well. When the rays of the mind are gathered and collected by practice, the mind becomes concentrated and you get Ananda from within. When you meet an old friend of yours after six years, the happiness you get is not, as is generally supposed from the friend, but from within yourself. The mind becomes concentrated for the time being and you get happiness from within your own self. The sum total of pleasures of the whole world is nothing when compared to the bliss derived through concentration and meditation. Do not give up the practice of concentration at any cost. Plod on. Have patience, perseverance, cheerfulness, tenacity and application. You will eventually succeed. *Nil desperandum.* Sri Sankaracharya writes in his commentary on the Chhandogya Upanishad: "A man's duty consists in the control of the senses and concentration of the mind." (Ch. VII-x-xii). Find out by serious introspection the various impediments that act as stumbling blocks in your concentration and remove them with effort one by one. Do not allow new thoughts (Sankalpas) and desires (Vasanas) to crop up. Nip them in the bud through discrimination, enquiry, concentration and meditation.

Everybody possesses some ability to concentrate. Everybody does concentrate to a certain extent when he reads a book, when he writes a letter, when he plays tennis and, in fact, when he does any kind of work. But for spiritual purposes concentration should be developed to an infinite degree. The mind is like an unchained monkey. It has the power of attending to one object only at a time, although it is able to pass from one object to another with tremendous speed, so rapidly, in fact, that some hold that it could grasp several things at a time. But the best philosophers and seers, Eastern and Western, hold to the "single idea" theory as being correct. It agrees with one's daily experience as well. The mind is ever restless. This is due to the force of Rajas or passion. Concentration is necessary for success in material affairs. A man with an appreciable degree of concentration has more earning capacity and turns out more work in less time. Need I say that the Yogic student will be amply rewarded for his effort in concentration?

When you study a book, focus your whole mind on the subject in hand. Do not allow the mind to see any external object or hear any sound. Collect all the dissipated rays of the mind. Develop the power of attention. Attention, as I have said somewhere in the beginning, plays no inconspicuous part in concentration. Concentration is, in fact, the narrowing of the field of attention. It is one of the signs of trained will. It is found in men of strong personality.

Practise attention on unpleasant tasks from which you have been shrinking on account of its unpleasantness. Throw interest upon uninteresting objects and ideas. Hold them on before your mind. Interest will slowly manifest. Many mental weaknesses will vanish. The mind will become stronger and stronger. The force wherewith anything strikes the mind is generally in proportion to the degree of attention bestowed upon it. Moreover, the great art of memory is attention and inattentive people have bad memories.

There is great concentration, when you play cards or chess, but the mind is not filled with pure and divine thoughts. The mental contents are of an undesirable nature. You can hardly experience the Divine Thrill, ecstasy and elevation of mind, when it is filled with impure thoughts. Every object has its own mental associations. You will have to fill up the mind with sublime spiritual thoughts. Then only the mind will be expurgated of all worldly thoughts. The picture of Lord Jesus or Buddha or Krishna is associated with sublime, soulstirring ideas; chess and cards are associated with ideas of gambling, cheating and so forth.

The invocation of shadow gives the objects seen as well as unseen. Undoubtedly a man becomes pure by its very sight. The shadow can also answer any question you may desire to ask. The Yogic practitioner who is able to see his own reflection in the sky will be able to know whether his undertakings will be crowned with success or not. Those Yogins who have realised the benefits of concentration fully have declared: "In a clear sunlit sky behold with a steady gaze your own reflection; whenever this is seen for a single second in the sky, you behold God at once in the sky." He who daily sees his shadow in the sky will acquire longevity. He will never meet with accidental death. When the shadow is seen fully reflected, then the Yogic practitioner gets victory and success. He conquers Prana and goes everywhere. The practice is simple enough. One realise the fruits in a short time. Some have realised the fruits in one or two weeks. When the sun rises, stand in such a way that your body casts a shadow upon the ground and you are able to see it without difficulty. Then steadily fix your gaze on the neck of the shadow for sometime and then look up into the sky. If you see a full grey shadow in the sky, it is very auspicious. The shadow will answer any question for you. If you do not get the shadow, continue the practice till you get it. You can practise this in the moonlight also.

Some people feel intense pain and agony when they suffer from some disease in some part of the body. The reason is not far to seek. They always think of the disease and do not know how to take the mind away from the affected part of the body by the practice of abstraction and fixing the mind on some other object. Some people feel less pain than others. Such people know how to divert the mind from the seat of disease. Whenever there is pain in the body, practise concentration on your tutelary deity or study some philosophical books. The pain will vanish.

Concentration is purely a mental process.[26] It needs an inward turning of the mind. It is not a muscular exercise. There should be no undue strain on the brain. You should not fight and wrestle with the mind violently.

Sit in a comfortable pose. Relax all the muscles of the body. There should neither be muscular nor emotional nor nervous nor mental strain. Keep a tight hold on the mental faculties. Still the mind. Silence the bubbling thoughts. Calm the emotions. Put a brake on the thought-process. Do not pay any attention to the intruding thoughts. Give the

26 For full particulars vide my book "*Sure Ways for success in Life and God-realisation*".

suggestion to the mind: "I do not care whether they are there or not." In other words, be indifferent. The intruding thoughts will quit the mental factory soon. They will not cause any trouble. This is the secret of mental discipline. Improvement in concentration will be visible only little by little. Do not be discouraged on any account. Be regular in your practice. Stop not the practice even for a single day. Lord Jesus says: "Empty thyself; I will fill thee." This process of emptying all thoughts should be attempted after you have attained some power of concentration. Keep yourself in a positive state always. When you wish to concentrate on a piece of work to be done with care, you can use all your will and imagination also. Imagination helps even concentration.

If you find it difficult to concentrate on the heart, on the tip of the nose, on the space between the eyebrows, or on the crown of the head, you can select any exernal object for the purpose. You can, for instance, concentrate on the blue sky, the light of the sun, the all-pervading air, ether, sun, moon, stars. If you experience any headache or pain in the skull or any part of the body due to the strain of concentration on a particular place or object, shift the centre of cancentration or change the object.

A Raja-Yogi concentrates on the space between the eyebrows (Ajna Chakra or Trikuti) which is the seat of the mind in the waking state. You can easily control the mind, if you concentrate on this region. Light is seen during concentration on this region very quickly. He who wants to meditate on the macrocosm (Virat) and he who wants to help the world should select this region for concentration. A

Bhakta or devotee should select the heart, the seat of emotion and feeling. He who concentrates on the heart gets immense happiness. He who wants to get something for himself should concentrate on the heart.

A scientist concentrates his mind and invents many things. Through concentration he opens the layers of the gross mind and penetrates deeply into higher regions of the mind and gets deeper knowledge. He concentrates all his energies into one focus and throws them upon the materials he is analysing, and so finds out their secrets. When there is faith, the mind can be easily concentrated on the subject to be understood; and then the understanding quickly follows. As mind evolves, you come into conscious relation with the mental currents, with the minds of others near and distant, living and dead. He who has learnt to manipulate the mind will get the whole nature under his control.

Too much physical exertion, too much talking, too much eating, too much mixing with ladies and undesirable persons, too much walking will cause distraction of mind. Those who practise concentration must abandon these things. Whatever work you do, do it with perfect concentration. Never leave the work without finishing it completely.

Celibacy, Pranayama, reduction of wants and activities, renunciation of objects, solitude, silence, discipline of the senses, annihilation of lust and greed, control of anger, non-mixing with undesirable persons, giving up of newspaper-reading-habit and visiting cinemas—all these pave a long way in increasing the power of concentratioln.

Even if the mind runs out during concentration, do not bother. Let it run. Slowly bring it to your object of concentration. In the beginning the mind may run 50 times, two years of practice will reduce the number to 20; another three years of continued and persistent practice will reduce the number to nil. The mind then will be completely fixed in the Divine consciousness. Then it will not run out even if you try to bring it out. This is the practical experience of those who have gained complete mastery over their minds.

Arjuna had wonderful concentration. He learnt the science of archery from Dronacharya. A dead bird was tied to a post in such a way that its reflection was cast in a basin of water right beneath on the ground. Arjuna saw the reflection of the bird in the basin of water and aimed successfully in hitting at the right eye of the actual bird tied to the post above.

Napoleon also had remarkable power of concentration. It is said that he had full control over his thoughts. He could draw one thought from a pigeon hole of his brain, dwell on that single thought as long as he liked and then shove that thought back into that pigeon-hole. He had a peculiar brain with peculiar pigeon-holes!

When you study a book with profound interest, you do not hear or see a man shouting or calling you by your name. You do not smell the sweet fragrance of flowers kept on the table by your side. This is concentration. This is one-pointedness of mind (Chitta-Ekagrata). The mind is fixed firmly on one thing and one thing only. Such must be the depth and intensity of your concentration, when you think of God or Atman. It is easy to concentrate the mind on worldly objects because the mind takes interest in it very naturally through force of habit. The grooves are already cut in the brain. You will have to create new grooves by fixing the mind again and again on God. After sometime the mind will not move to external objects, for it experiences joy and bliss within.

Some Western psychologists hold: "The mind that wanders aimlessly can be made to move in a small limited circle only, by the practice of concentration. It cannot be fixed on one point only. If it is fixed on one point only, then inhibition of the mind will take place. There is death for the mind. Nothing can be achieved when there is inhibition of the mind. So there is no use of inhibiting the mind." This is not right. Complete control of the mind can be attained, when all the thought-waves are extirpated thoroughly. The Yogi works wonders by his one-pointedness of mind. He knows the hidden treasures of the Soul with the help of the mighty all-penetrating search-light generated by the one-pointedness of mind. Afer one-pointedness (Ekagrata) is attained, you have to achieve full restraint (Nirodha). In this state all modifications subside completely. The mind becomes quite blank. Then the Yogi destroys this blank mind also by identifying himself with the Supreme Purusha or Soul or Being from whom the mind borrows its light. Then he obtains Omniscience and final emancipation (Kaivalya). These are matters that are Greek and Latin to our Western psychologists. Hence they grope in darkness. They have no idea of the Purusha who witnesses the activities of the mind.

Man is a complex social animal. He is a biological organism and so he is definitely characterised by the possession of certain physiological functions such as circulation of blood, digestion, respiration, excretion, etc. He is also definitely characterised by the possession of certain psychological functions such as thinking, perception, memory, imagination, etc. He sees, thinks, tates, smells and feels. Philosophically speaking, he is the image of God, nay he is God himself. He lost his divine glory by tasting the fruit of the forbidden tree. He can regain his lost divinity by mental discipline and the practice of concentration.

## EXERCISES

### I

Ask your friend to show you some playing cards. Immediately after the exposure, describe the forms you have seen. Give the number, name, etc., such as club king, spade ten, diamond queen, heart jack, and so on.

### II

Read two or three pages of a book. Then close the book. Now attend to what you have read. Abandon all distracting thoughts. Focus your attention carefully. Allow the mind to associate, classify, group, combine and compare. You will get now a fund of knowledge and information on the subject. Mere skipping over the pages inadvertently is of no use. There are students who read a book within a few hours. If you ask them to reproduce some important points of the book, they will simply blink. If you attend to the subject on hand very carefully, you will receive clear, strong impressions. If the impressions are strong, you will have very good memory.

### III

Sit on your favourite meditative pose about one foot from a watch. Concentrate on the *tik-tik* sound slowly. Whenever the mind runs, again and again try to hear the sound. Just see how long the mind can be fixed continuously on the sound.

### IV

Sit again on your favourite Asana. Close your eyes. Close the ears with your thumbs or plug the ears with wax or cotton. Try to hear the Anahata sounds (mystic sounds). You will hear various kinds of sounds such as flute, violin, kettledrum, thunder-storm, conch, bells, the humming of a bee, etc. Try to hear the gross sounds first. Hear only one kind of sound. If the mind runs, you can shift it from gross to subtle, or from subtle to gross. Generally you will hear sounds in your right ear. Occasionally you may hear in your left ear also. But try to stick to the sound of one ear. You will get one-pointedness of mind. This is an easy way to capture the mind, because it is enchanted by the sweet sound just as a snake is hypnotised by the note of the snake-charmer.

Keep a candle-flame in front of you and try to concentrate on the flame. When you are tired of doing this, close your eyes and try to visualise the flame. Do it for half a minute and increase the time to five or ten minutes according to your taste, temperament and capacity. You will see Rishis and Devatas, when you enter into deep concentration.

### VI

In a lying posture, concentrate on the moon. Whenever the mind runs, again and again bring it back to the image of the moon. This exercise is very beneficial in the case of some persons having an emotional temperament.

## VII

In the above manner, you can concentrate on any star you may single out from the millions of stars, shining above your head.

## VIII

Sit by the side of a river where you can hear a roaring sound like OM. Concentrate on that sound as long as you like. This is very thrilling and inspiring.

## IX

Lie on your bed in the open air and concentrate upon the blue expansive sky above. Your mind will expand immediately. You will be elevated. The blue sky will remind you of the infinite nature of the Self.

Sit in a comfortable posture and concentrate on any one of the numerous abstract virtues such as mercy. Dwell upon this virtue as long as you can.

## Lesson IX

# MEDITATION

**M**editation follows concentration. Concentration merges into meditation. Concentration is holding the mind on to some particular object. An unbroken flow of knowledge in that subject is meditation. Meditation is regular flow of thought with regard to the object of concentration. Meditation opens the door of the mind to intuitive knowledge and many powers. You can get whatever you want through meditation. During meditation all worldly thoughts are shut out from the mind. Meditation is called *Dhyana* in Sanskrit and is the seventh step in the Yogic ladder.

In Lesson VII you were advised to keep a separate room for practising Pranayama, isn't it so? Well, the same room will also serve the purpose of meditation. In fact, one room will be quite sufficient for all spiritual practices—Asanas, Pranayama, Japa,[27] Kirtan,[28] concentration, meditation, and so forth. The room should be regarded as a temple of God. You should not allow anybody into the room. You should enter the room with a pious and reverent mind. Thoughts of jealousy, lust, greed

---

27 *Twirling the beads along with the repetition of a Mantra.*
28 *Singing the Names of the Lord or other devotional songs.*

and anger should not be entertained within the four walls of the room. All worldly talks, also should not be indulged in there. For every word that is uttered, every thought that is cherished and every deed that is done is not lost; they are reflected on the subtle layers of ether encircling the room where they are done and hence affect the mind invariably.

Decorate the room with inspiring pictures of great Saints, Sages, Prophets and World Teachers. In a prominent place in the room keep a beautiful photo of your tutelary Deity (Ishta-Devata), either Lord Jesus, Lord Krishna, Lord Siva or Devi. Let the Deity face the East or North. Spread your Asana (seat) in front of the Deity. Keep some religious and philosophical books such as the Bhagavadgita, the Upanishads, the Vedanta-Sutras, the Ramayana, the Yoga-Vasishtha, the Bible, etc., by your side. Wash your face, hands and legs before you enter the room. Burn a piece of camphor and light some scented sticks immediately after entering the room. Sit on the Asana in front of the Deity and repeat the Name of the Lord or sing some devotional hymns. Then take to the practice of concentration and meditation.

Of course, even if you wander from pole to pole, you cannot get an ideal place that will satisfy you from every standpoint. Every place has some advantages and some disadvantages as well. So you should select a place that is more advantageous than others. Having once hit upon a place, you must stick to it till the last. You must not think of changing the place, when some difficulty stares you in the face. You must put up with the difficulty by all means. Rishikesh (Himalayas), Haridwar, Uttarkashi,

Badrinarayan, Gangotri, Mount Kailas, Brindavan, Varanasi, Nasik and Ayodhya are all excellent places for meditation in India.

The best and the most congenial time for the practice of meditation is unquestionably the *Brahmamuhurta* i.e., from 4 to 6 a.m. That is the time when the mind is quite refreshed after an agreeable slumber, when the mind is calm and comparatively pure. It is like a clean blank sheet of paper. Only such a mind can be moulded into whatever shape you like. Moreover, the atmosphere also is charged with purity and goodness at this time.

In the beginning you can meditate twice daily, frorn 4 to 5 in the morning and 7 to 8 at night. As you advance in your practices, you can increase the duration of each sitting little by little using your commonsense and discretion, and also have a third sitting either in the morning between 10 and 11 or in the evening between 4 and 5.

In the Yoga-Vasishtha you will find: "The right course to be adopted by one who is in his novitiate is this: Two parts of the mind must be filled with the objects of Enjoyment, one part with Philosophy and the remaining part with Devotion to the teacher. Having advanced a little, he should fill one part of the mind with the objects of Enjoyment, two parts with Devotion to the teacher and the remaining one with getting an insight into the meaning of Philosophy. When one has attained proficiency, he should everyday fill two parts of his mind with Philosophy and supreme Renunciation, and the remaining two parts with Meditation and devoted Service to the Guru." This will eventually lead you on to meditation for twenty-four hours.

Sitting on your favourite meditative pose and keeping the head, neck and trunk erect, close your eyes and gently concentrate on either the tip of the nose, space between the eyebrows, the heart-lotus or the crown of the head. When once you have selected one centre of concentration, stick to it till the last with leech-like tenacity. Never change it. Thus, if you have chosen to concentrate on the heart-lotus after having tried the other centres, stick to the heart-lotus alone. Then only you can expect rapid advancement.

Meditation is of two kinds viz., Saguna (with Gunas or qualities) meditation and Nirguna (without Gunas or qualities) meditation. Meditation on Lord Krishna, Lord Siva, Lord Rama or Lord Jesus is Saguna meditation. It is meditation with form and attributes. The Name of the Lord is also simultaneously repeated. This is the method of the Bhaktas. Meditation on the reality of the Self is Nirguna meditation. This is the method of the Vedantins. Meditation on *Om, Soham, Sivoham, Aham Brahma Asmi* and *Tat Tvam Asi* is Nirguna meditation.

Put an iron rod in the blazing furnace. It becomes red like fire. Remove it from the fire. It loses its red colour. If you want to keep it always red, you must keep it always in fire. Even so, if you want to keep the mind charged with the fire of Brahmic Wisdom, you must keep it always in contact with the Brahmic Fire of Knowledge through constant and intense meditation. You must, in other words, keep up an unceasing flow of Brahmic Consciousness.

Meditation is the most powerful mental and nervine tonic. The holy vibrations penetrate all the cells of the body and cure the various diseases that human flesh is heir to.

Those who regularly meditate save the doctor's bills. The powerful soothing waves that arise during meditation exercise a benign influence on the mind, nerves, organs and cells of the body. The divine energy freely flows like the flow of oil from one vessel to another, from the Feet of the Lord to the different systems of the practitioner.

If you meditate for half an hour, you will be able to face the daily battle of life with peace and spiritual strength for one week through the force of meditation. Such is the beneficial effect of meditation. As you have to move with different minds of peculiar nature, get the requisite strength and peace from meditation and be free from worry and trouble.

The wise cut asunder the knot of egoism by the sharp sword of constant meditation. Then dawns supreme Knowledge of the Self or full Illumination or Self-realisation. The liberated sage has neither doubt nor delusion. All bonds of Karma (action) are rent asunder. Therefore be ever engaged in meditation. This is the master-key to open the realms of eternal Bliss. It may be disgusting and tiring in the beginning, because the mind will be running away from the point (Lakshya) every now and then. But after sometime it will be focussed in the centre. You will be immersed in Divine Bliss.

Regular meditation opens up the avenues of intuitional knowledge, makes the mind calm and steady, awakens an ecstatic feeling, and brings the Yogic student in contact with the Supreme Purusha. If there are doubts, they are all cleared by themselves, when you march on the path of Dhyana-Yoga (meditation) steadily. You will yourself feel

the way to place your footstep in the next higher rung of the
Yogic ladder. A mysterious inner voice will guide you.
Hear thou this attentively, O Yogananda!

When you get a flash of illumination, do not be
frightened. It will be a new experience of immense joy. Do
not turn back. Do not give up meditation. Do not stop there.
You will have to advance still further. This is only a
glimpse of truth. This is not the whole experience. This is
not the highest realisation. This is only a new platform. Try
to ascend further. Reach the Bhuma or the Infinite. Now
alone you are proof against all temptations. You will drink
deep the nectar of Immortality. This is the acme or final
stage. You can take eternal rest now. You need not meditate
any further. This is the final goal.

You have within yourself tremendous powers and
latent faculties of which you have really never had any
conception. You must awaken these dormant powers and
faculties by the practice of meditation and Yoga. You must
develop your will and control your senses and mind. You
must purify yourself and practise regular meditation. Then
only you can become a Superman or God-man.

There is no such thing as miracle or Siddhi. Ordinary
man is quite ignorant of higher spiritual things. He is sunk
in oblivion. He is shut up from higher transcendental
knowledge. So he calls some extraordinary event a miracle.
But for a Yogi who understands things in the light of Yoga,
there is no such thing as miracle. Just as a villager is
astonished at the sight of an aeroplane or a talkie for the
first time, so also a man of the world is stunned when he
sees an extraordinary spectacle for the first time.

Every human being has within himself various potentialities and capacities. He is a magazine of power and knowledge. As he evolves, he unfolds new powers, new faculties, new qualities. Now he can change his environments and influence others. He can subdue other minds. He can conquer internal and external nature. He can enter into super-conscious state.

In a dark room if a pot containing a lamp inside it, is broken, the darkness of the room is dispelled and you see light everywhere in the room. Even so, if the body-pot is broken through constant meditation on the Self, i.e., if you destroy ignorance (Avidya) and its effects such as identification with the body, and rise above body-consciousness, you will cognise the supreme light of the Atman everywhere.

Just as the water in the pot that is placed in the ocean becomes one with the waters of the ocean, when the pot is broken, so also when the body-pot is broken by meditation on the Atman, the individual soul becomes one with the Supreme Soul.

Just as the light is burning within the hurricane lamp, so also the Divine Flame is burning from time immemorial in the lamp of your heart. Close your eyes. Merge youself within the Divine Flame. Plunge deep into the chambers of your heart. Meditate on this Divine Flame and become one with the Flame of God.

If the wick within the lamp is small the light will also be small. If the wick is big, the light also will be powerful. Similarly, if the Jiva (individual soul) is pure, if he practises meditation, the manifestation or expression of the Self will be powerful. He will radiate a big light. If he is unregenerate and impure, he will be like a burnt-up charcoal. The bigger the wick, the greater the light. Likewise, the purer the soul, the greater the expression.

If the magnet is powerful, it will influence the iron filings even when they are placed at a distance. Even so, if the Yogi is an advanced person, he will have greater influence over the persons with whom he comes in contact. He can exert his influence on persons even when they live in distant places.

The fire of meditation annihilates all foulness due to viee. Then suddenly there comes Knowledge of Self or Divine Wisdom which directly lends to Mukti or final emancipation.

During meditation note how long you can shut out all worldly thoughts. Watch your mind. If it is for twenty minutes, try to increase the period to thirty minutes and so on. Fill the mind with thoughts of God again and again.

In meditation do not strain your eyes. Do not strain the brain. Do not struggle or wrestle with the mind. Relax. Gently allow the divine thoughts to flow. Steadily think of the Lakshya (point of meditation). Do not voluntarily and violently drive away the intruding thoughts. Have sublime Sattvic thoughts. The vicious thoughts will by themselves vanish.

If there is much strain in your meditation, reduce the duration of each sitting for a few days. Do light meditation only. When you have regained the normal tone, again increase the period. Use your common-sense throughout your Sadhana. I always reiterate on this point.

"Though men should perform Tapas standing on one leg for a period of 1,000 years, it will not in the least, be equal to one-sixteenth part of Dhyana-Yoga (meditation)." *Pingala-Upanishad.*

Those who meditate for four or five hours at a stretch can have two meditative poses. Sometimes the blood accumulates in one part of the legs or thighs and so gives a little trouble. After two hours change the pose. Or stretch the legs at full length and lean against a wall or pillow. Keep the spine erect. This is the most comfortable Asana. Or join two chairs. Sit in one chair and stretch the legs on another chair. This is another contrivance.

You must daily increase your Vairagya, meditation and Sattvic virtues such as patience, perseverance, mercy, love, forgiveness, etc. Vairagya and good qualities help meditation. Meditation increases the Sattvic qualities.

Considerable changes take place in the mind, brain and the nervous system by the practice of meditation. New nerve-currents, new vibrations, new avenues, new grooves, new cells, new channels are formed. The whole mind and the nervous system are remodelled. You will have a new heart, a new mind, new sensations, new feelings, new mode of thinking and acting and a new view of the universe (as God in manifestation).

During meditation you will get into rapture or ecstasy. It is of five kinds viz., the lesser thrill, momentary rapture, flooding rapture, transporting rapture, and all-pervading rapture. The lesser thrill will raise the hairs of the body (like the goose-skin). The momentary rapture is like the productions of lightning moment by moment. Like waves breaking on the seashore, the flooding rapture descends rapidly on the body and breaks. Transporting rapture is strong and lifts the body up to the extent of launching it into the air. When the all-pervading rapture arises, the whole body is completely surcharged and blown like a full bladder.

"Whatever he (the Yogic practitioner) sees with his eyes, let him consider as Atman. Whatever he hears with his ears, let him consider as Atman. Whatever he smells with his nose, let him consider as Atman. Whatever he tastes with his tongue, let him consider as Atman. Whatever the Yogi touches with his skin, let him consider as Atman. The Yogi should thus unwearied gratify his organs of sense for a period of one Yama (3 hours) every day with great effort. The various wonderful powers are attained by the Yogi, such as clairvoyance, clairaudience, ability to transport himself to great distances within a moment, great power of speech, ability to take any form, ability to become invisible, and the transmutation of iron into gold, when the former is smeared over with his excretion." *Yogatattva-Upanishad.*

Just as a very skilful archer in shooting at a bird is aware of the way in which he takes his steps, holds the bow, the bow-string, and the arrow at the time when he pierces the bird, thus "standing in this position, holding thus the bow, thus the bow-string, and thus the arrow, I pierce the bird," and ever afterwards would not fail to fulfil these conditions that he might pierce the bird, even so the aspirant should note the conditions such as suitable food, thus "eating this kind of food, following such a person, in such a dwelling in this mode, at this time, I attained to this meditation and Samadhi."

As a clever cook in serving his master notes the kind of food that his master relishes and henceforward serves it and gets gain, so the aspirant too notes the conditions such as nourishment, etc., at the moment of attaining meditation and Samadhi and in fulfilling them gets ecstasy again and again.

Leading a virtuous life is not by itself sufficient for God-realisation. Concentration of mind is absolutely necessary. A good virtuous life only prepares the mind as a fit instrument for concentration and meditation. It is concentration and meditation that eventually lead to Self-realisation or God-realisation.

"A Yogi should always avoid fear, anger, laziness, too much sleep or waking and too much food and fasting. If the above rule he well and strictly practised each day, spiritual wisdom will arise of itself in three months without doubt. In four months, he sees the Devatas; in five months, he knows (or becomes) Brahmanishtha; and in six months, he attains Kaivalya at will. There is no doubt." *Amritananda-Upanishad.*

During meditation some of the visions that you see are your own materialised thoughts, while some others are real objective visions. In meditation new grooves are formed in the brain and the mind moves upwards in the new spiritual grooves. In meditation and concentration you will have to train the, mind in a variety of ways. Then only the gross mind will become subtle.

When you first practise meditation, lights of various colours such as red, white, blue, green and a mixture of red and green, etc., will appear in the forehead. These are Tanmatric (elemental) lights. Every element has got its own colour. Water has white colour. Fire has red colour. Air has green colour. Ether has blue colour. So the colourful lights are due to these Tattvas (elements) only.

Some times you may see a big blazing sun or moon or lightning in front of the forehead. Do not mind these. Shun them. Try to dive deep into the source of these lights.

Sometimes Devatas, Nitya Siddhas (eternally perfected Yogins) and Amarapurushas (immortal beings) will appear in meditation. Receive them all with due honour. Bow down before them. Get advice from them. Do not be frightened. They appear before you to give you all spiritual help and encouragement.[29]

"Having made Atman as the lower Arani (sacrificial wood) and the Pranava as the upper Arani, one should see the God in secret through the practice of churning which is Dhyana (meditation)." *Dhyanabindu-Upanishad.*

---

[29] For further particulars vide my book "*Paractice of Yoga*".

## EXERCISES

### I

Place a picture of Lord Jesus in front of you. Sit in your favourite meditative pose. Concentrate gently with open eyes on the picture till tears trickle down your cheeks. Rotate the mind on the cross, on the chest, long hairs, beautiful beard, round eyes, and the various other limbs of his body; the fine spiritual aura emanating from his head, and so on. Think of his divine attributes such as love, magnanimity, mercy and forbearance. Think of the various phases of his interesting life and the "miracles" he performed and the various "extraordinary" powers he possessed. Then close your eyes and try to visualise the picture. Repeat the same process again and again.

### II

Place a picture of Lord Hari in front of you. Sit again in your meditative posture. Concentrate gently on the picture till you shed tears. Rotate the mind on His feet, legs, yellow silken robes, golden garland set with diamonds, Koustubha gem, etc., on the chest, the earrings, then the face, the crown of the head, the disc on the right upper hand, the conch on the left upper hand, the mace on the right lower hand, and the lotus-flower on the left lower hand. Then close the eyes and try to visualise the picture. Repeat the same process again and again.

### III

Keep a picture of Lord Krishna with flute in hands in front of you. Sit in your meditative pose and gently concentrate on the picture till you shed tears. Think of His feet adorned with anklets, yellow garment, various ornaments round His neck, the necklace set with the

Koustubha gem, the long garland of beautiful flowers of various colours, ear-rings, crown set with precious jewels of priceless value, dark and long hairs, sparkling eyes, the Tilaka[30] on the forehead, the magnetic aura round His head, long hands adorned with bracelets and armlets, and the flute in the hands ready to be played upon. Then close your eyes and visualise the picture. Repeat the same process again and again.

## IV

This is one kind of meditation for beginners. Sit on Padmasana in your meditation room. Close your eyes. Meditate on the effulgence in the sun, or the splendour in the moon or the glory in the stars.

## V

Meditate on the magnanimity of the ocean and its infinite nature. Then compare the ocean to the Infinite Brahman, and the waves, foams and ice-bergs to the various names and forms. Identify yourself with the ocean. Become silent. Expand. Expand.

## VI

This is another kind of meditation. Meditate on the Himalayas. Imagine that the Ganga takes its origin in the icy regions of Gangotri near Uttarakasi, flows through Rishikesh, Haridwar, Benares, and then enters into the Bay of Bengal near Gangasagar. Himalayas, Ganga and the sea—these three thoughts only should occupy your mind. First take your mind to the icy regions of Gangotri, then

30Mark or symbol made with sandalwood or ungent

along the Ganga and finally to the sea. Rotate the mind in this manner for 10 minutes.

### VII

There is a living Universal Power that underlies all these names and forms. Meditate on this Power which is formless. This will terminate in the realisation of the Absolute, Nirguna, Nirakara (formless) Consciousness eventually.

### VIII

Sit on Padmasana. Close your eyes. Gaze steadily on the formless air only. Concentrate on the air. Meditate on the all-pervading nature of the air. This will lead to the realisation of the nameless and formless Brahman, the One Living Truth.

### IX

Sit on your meditative pose. Close your eyes. Imagine that there is a supreme, infinite effulgence hidden behind all these names and forms which is tantamount to the effulgence of crores of suns put together. This is another form of Nirguna meditation.

### X

Concentrate and meditate on the expansive blue sky. This is another kind of Nirguna meditation. By the previous methods of concentration the mind will cease thinking of finite forms. It will slowly begin to melt in the ocean of Peace, as it is deprived of its contents. The mind will become subtler and subtler.

### XI

Have the picture of OM in front of you. Concentrate gently on this picture with open eyes till tears flow profusely. Associate the ideas of eternity, infinity, immortality, etc., when you think of OM. The humming of bees, the sweet notes of the nightingale, the seven tunes in music, and all sounds are emanating from OM only. OM is the essence of the Vedas. Imagine that OM is the bow, the mind is the arrow and Brahman (God) is the target. Aim at the target with great care and then, like the arrow becomes one with the target, you will become one with Brahman. The short accent of OM burns all sins, the long accent gives Moksha, and the elongated accent bestows all psychic powers (Siddhis). He who chants and meditates upon this monosyllable OM chants and meditates upon all the Scriptures of the world.

## XII

Sit on Padmasana or Siddhasana in your meditation room. Watch the flow of breath. You will hear the sound *"SOHAM"*, So during inhalation and *ham* during exhalation. SOHAM means I AM HE. The breath is reminding you of your identity with the Supreme Soul. You are unconsciously repeating Soham 21,600 times daily at the rate of 15 Sohams per minute. Associate the ideas of Existence, Knowledge, Bliss, Absolute, Purity, Peace, Perfection, Love, etc., along with Soham. Negate the body while repeating the Mantra and identify yourself with the Atman or the Supreme Soul.

## XIII

Uddhava asked Lord Krishna: "O Lotus-eyed! How to meditate on Thee! Tell me what is the nature of that meditation and what it is?" To which Lord Krishna replied: "Be seated on the Asana that is neither high nor low, with your body erect and in an easy posture. Place your hands on the lap. Fix your gaze on the tip of the nose (in order to fix the mind). Purify the tracks of Prana by Puraka, Kumbhaka and Rechaka, and then again in the reverse way i.e., first breathe in by the left nostril with the right nostril closed by the tip of the thumb, then close the left nostril by the tips of the ring finger and the little finger and retain the breath in both the nostrils. Then remove the tip of the thumb and breathe out through the right nostril. Reverse the process by breathing in through the right nostril, then retaining the breath in both the nostrils and letting out the breath through the left nostril. Practise this Pranayama gradually with your senses controlled.

"Aum" with the sound of a bell, extends all over, from Muladhara[31] upwards. Raise the "Aum" in the heart by means of Prana (twelve fingers upwards) as if it were the thread of a lotus-stalk. There let Bindu (the fifteenth vowel sound) be added to it. Thus practise Pranayama accompanied by the Pranava reciting the latter ten times. Continue the practice, three times a day, and within a month you shall be able to control the vital air. The lotus of the heart has its stalk upwards and the flower downwards, facing below (and it is also closed, like the inflorescence with bracts of the banana *Sridhara*). Meditate on it, however, as facing upwards and full-blown, with eight petals and with the pericap. On the pericap, think of the sun, the moon, and fire one after another. First meditate on all the limbs. Then let the mind withdraw the senses from their objects. Then draw the concentrated mind completely towards Me, by means of Buddhi (intellect). Then give up

31 *See Lesson XI*

all other limbs and concentrate on one thing only, My smiling face. Do not meditate on anything else. Then withdraw the concentrated mind from that and fix it on the Akasa (ether). Give up that also and being fixed in Me (as Brahman) think of nothing at all. You shall see Me in Atman, as identical with all Atmans, even as light is identical with another light. The delusions about objects, knowledge and action shall then completely disappear. This is a beautiful exercise for meditation prescribed by Lord Krishna Himself in the Bhagavata Purana.

## SAMADHI

*"Which, having obtained, he thinketh there is no greater gain beyond it; wherein, established, he is not shaken even by heavy sorrow."*—Bhagavad-Gita: Ch. VI-22

The fruit of meditation is Samadhi. Samadhi is super conscious state, wherein the Yogi gets superintuitional or supersensual knowledge and Supersensual bliss. He gets the vision of the Lord. He is in a state of communion with the Lord. He is in full enjoyment of the Divine Ecstasy or Divine Thrill. He has seen the Light of lights now.

The five afflictions, reference to which was made in Lesson I, have now come to an end. All sorts of imperfections have disappeared. Just as the river has joined the sea, the individual soul has joined the Supreme Soul. All limitations have dropped now. This state cannot be described in words: It has to he felt by actual practice. There are neither wants nor desires here. All doubts and delusions, all sorrows and tribulations, all fears, differences, distinctions and dualities have vanished entirely. This is the ultimate goal of all spiritual practices. This is the goal of life.

Samadhi is the eighth step of the Yogic ladder. Intuition, revelation, inspiration and ecstasy are all synonymous terms. The meditator and the meditated, the thinker and the thought, the worshipper and the worshipped, the subject and the object have now become identical. The meditator has merged himself in the Soul or the all-pervading Spirit. All watertight compartments have disappeared. The Yogi feels oneness and unity everywhere. He feels: "I have nothing more to learn. I have nothing more to do. I have nothing more to obtain."

That which is night of all beings is the time of waking for the illumined Yogi; when other beings are waking, then it is night for him. Yajnavalkya, the greatest Yogi says: "By Pranayama impurities of the body are destroyed; by Dharana or concentration impurities of the mind. By Pratyahara the impurities of attachment and by Samadhi everything that hides the Soul is removed."

Samadhi is of two kinds viz., *Savikalpa* Samadhi and *Nirvikalpa* Samadhi. Savikalpa is a lower Samadhi. In the Savikalpa Samadhi the Samskaras or latent impressions are not fried *in toto*. There is support for the mind. There is still the triad of subtle type viz., the seer, sight and seen, or the knower, knowledge and knowable. So Savikalpa Samadhi cannot give full satisfaction, full freedom, full bliss and knowledge.

In Nirvikalpa Samadhi all Samskaras are burnt *in toto*. There is no support for the mind. The mind has merged into the all-pervading Spirit. There is no triad of seer, sight and seen, and so forth. Nirvikalpa Samadhi gives full satisfaction, full freedom, full bliss and full knowledge.

There is also another classification viz., *Jada* Samadhi and *Chaitanya* Samadhi. In Jada Samadhi there is no awareness. It is more or less like deep sleep. The Yogi does not return with intuitional knowledge. The Samskaras and desires are not destroyed. This is the Samadhi of the Hatha-Yogins who practise Khechari Mudra.[32] Somehow the Prana is fixed in some lower Chakra or centre of spiritual energy, and the Yogi remains like a dead corpse. The Yogi can even be buried in a box underneath the ground for several days at a stretch. Jada Samadhi cannot give liberation or Mukti. It is more like an acrobatic feat. The Samadhi that we often hear of persons entering into, in public places is nothing but Jada Samadhi. In the other variety of Samadhi viz.. Chaitanya Samadhi, there is *"perfect awareness."* The Yogi has intuitional knowledge.

William Wordsworth, the great English poet, describes Samadhi as follows:—

"....That blessed mood,
In which the burthen of the mystery,
In which the heavy and the weary weight
Of all this unintelligible world,
Is lightened—That serene and blessed mood,
In which the affections gently lead us on,
Until the breath of this corporeal frame
And even the motion of our human blood
Almost suspended, we are laid asleep
In body, and become a living soul;
While with an eye made quiet by the power

---

32 *Reversing the tongue backwards and upwards, fixing it at the root of the palate and closing up the posterior nasal openings is Khechari Mudra.*

Of harmony, and the deep power of joy,
We see into the life of things."

Sankara, Dattatreya, Vamadeva, Jada Bharata, Madalasa and Yajnavalkya had all the experience of supercosmic consciousness (Nirvikalpa Samadhi), while Ramadas, Tulasidas, Kabir, Tukaram, Mira, Gouranga, Hafiz, Madhva and Ramanuja had the experience of cosmic consciousness (Savikalpa Samadhi). Dr. Maurice Bucke, the celebrated author of "Cosmic Consciousness" believes that St. John of the Cross, Bacon, Jacob Behman, Pascal, Spinoza, Swedenborg. William Wordsworth, Alexander Pushkin, Honore de Balzac, Emerson, Tennyson, Thoreau, Walt Whitman and Edward Carpenter had the good fortune to taste the nectar of cosmic consciousness. As a Hindu example he also mentions the name of Ramakrishna Paramahamsa of Bengal.

He who poses for a great Yogi before the public and advertises in newspapers that at such and such time on such and such day he is going to enter into Samadhi does so with a view to make money and also a name for himself. He is actually deceiving and swindling the public in broad daylight. A real Yogi who has reached the goal of life and is always in Samadhi throughout the twenty-four hours will never make a parade of his attainment. He will never even tell others that he is enjoying the bliss of Samadhi. It is only the empty drum that maketh much sound.

In the waking state you do conscious work, but you are not conscious of the working of the heart, stomach, liver, etc. Just as there is unconscious work beneath the level of objective consciousness, so also there is superconsciousness above the level of physical consciousness, wherein there is play of neither the mind nor the senses. The man who returns from sleep does not possess any new knowledge, whereas he who comes down from Samadhi possesses supersensual knowledge. He can clear any doubt concerning the problems of life.

'The Yogin is one who has realised the Brahman that is all-full beyond Turiya[33] They (the people) extol him as Brahman; and becoming the object of the praise of the whole world, he wanders over different countries....Then the Yogin becomes immersed in the ocean of bliss. When compared to it, the bliss of Indra and others is very little. He who gets this bliss is the supreme Yogin." *Mandalabrahrnana-Upanishad)* .

Again in the Yogatattva-Upanishad it is said: "One who is engaged in Nirguna Dhyana attains the stage of Samadhi. Within twelve days at least, he attains the stage of Samadhi. Restraining the breath, the wise one becomes an emancipated person. Samadhi is that state in which the Jivatman (Lower Self) and the Paramatman (Higher Self) are differenceless (or of equal state). If he desires to lay aside his body, he can do so....But if he does not so desire, and if his body is dear to him, he lives in all the worlds possessing the Siddhis of Anima, etc. Sometimes he becomes a Deva and lives honoured in Svarga; or he becomes a man or a Yaksha through will. He can also take

---

33 *There are four states of consciousness viz., waking (Jagrat) state, dreaming (Svapna) state deep sleep (Sushupti) state, and superconscious (Turiya) state. There is a state still higher, or rather the highest of all, and that is Turiyateeta state. In this state the Jivatman gets absorbed into Brahman. This is the goal of life.*

the form of a lion, tiger, elephant, or horse through his own will. The Yogin becoming the great Lord can live as long as he likes."

The word Samyama is used in Yogic literature to denote the triple process of concentration, meditation and Samadhi practised at one and the same time. The Yogi acquires various powers by practising this Samyama. Samyama on the three kinds of changes viz., of form, time and state gives knowledge of the past and the future. Samyama on word, meaning and knowledge bestows knowledge of all animal sounds. One acquires the knowledge of life by perceiving the impressions. Samyama on the signs of another's body (such as the complexion, voice, mole, or any such sign on the body) reveals the knowledge of your own mind. Samyama on friendship, mercy, and love enables you to excel others in those qualities. Samyama on the strength of an elephant and others gives you their respective strength. Samyama on the navel circle gives you the knowledge of the constitution of your body. By doing Samyama on the light emanating from the top of the head (during concentration and meditation) you will acquire the power of beholding the Siddhas (perfected sages). You will also get clairvoyance, clairaudience, thought-reading, and so forth.

Patanjali Maharshi, the holy Author of the "Yoga-Sutras" gives a definite warning to the students of Yoga in this connection. He remarks that though these are the accompaniments of the outgoing mind, they are all obstacles to feel Samadhi. The real Yogi will reject these powers ruthlessly. The seeds of bondage can be destroyed only by non-attachment and dispassion. Then only you can attain Kaivalya or Absolute Independence. These Siddhis are, no doubt, very tempting and alluring. Many Yogic students get deluded. They become slaves of these powers. Consequently they get a downfall. They become stranded. They are not able to march onwards and reach the goal. The real Yogi marches on towards the goal fearlessly. His aim is the attainment of the glorious Freedom or the state of Asamprajnata Samadhi (same as Nirvikalpa Samadhi), wherein all the seeds of actions are burnt. He therefore shines in his active Effulgence of eternal life and full illumination and perfection.

There is an interesting story in the Yoga-Vasishtha illustrating the bliss of Samadhi. Kacha, the son of Brihaspati, the priest of the Devas, came out from his Samadhi with a cheerful mind, and soliloquised thus, in words bubbling with emotion: "What shall I do, where shall I go, what shall I take and what shall I give up? The whole universe is filled with the Self, as if with the waters of the Great Deluge. Within and without the body, below, above, and at all points of the compass, here, there and everywhere, is the Self; there is no spot filled with the not-self anywhere. There is nothing wherein I do not abide, nor is there anything which is not in me. What else shall I desire, when everything is pervaded by the Supreme Consciousness! The seven mountain fabled to hold up the globe of this earth are but the foam over the waters of this vast, mighty and pure ocean of the all-pervading Brahman. Before the great radiance of the Sun of this Supreme Consciousness, all the wealth and glory of the world are but so many mirages."

The Trance of Prahlada also illustrates in an equally illuminating and thrilling manner the glory of Samadhi. Wrapt in his thought, Prahlada lost himself in the Supreme Bliss of Ecstatic Trance. While remaining in this blessed condition, he appeared, as it were, a mere picture or statue of his painted on a canvas. He continued in this state with body ever fresh and bright and with his eyes filled on one point, for a period of five thousand years. "Awake, ye great soul!"—addressing thus, the Lord Vishnu blew His conch Panchajanya, filling the quarters with the echo of its sound. By the impact of this mighty sound, generated by the vital breath of Vishnu, the Lord of the Asuras (demons) was awakened, by slow degrees, to the life of the world.

And then the story of Sikhidhvaja is most awe-inspiring of all! Chudalai, the queen of Sikhidhvaja, saw her lord immersed in the thought-suppressed variety of trance and thought within herself; "Let me rouse my lord, the King, from this state of Ecstasy." So saying, she roared mightily like a lion, over and over, frightening the beasts of the forest. When he could not be moved by this terrible noise though frequently repeated, she shook him out of the trance by physical force. But, though thus shaken and felled to the ground, the King would not awake to the life of the ordinary world!

When the Purusha is thus completely disconnected from the three Gunas and their effects, when he has realised his own pristine glory, Isolation of Absolute Independence, and when he feels his Absolute Freedom, then alone he attains Kaivalya, the highest goal of a Yogi. The past and the future are now blended into the "PRESENT." Everything is "NOW and HERE" for him. The sum total of all knowledge of the three worlds is nothing when compared to the Infinite Knowledge of a Yogi who has attained Kaivalya. Glory unto such blessed Yogins! May their blessings be upon us all![34]

---

34 *For further details and particulars refer to my book "Practice of Bhakti-Yoga."*

*Lesson XI*

## THE SERPENTINE POWERS

The Serpentine Power is called Kundalini-Sakti on account of its spiral-like working in the body of the Yogi developing the power in himself. It is an electric fiery occult power, the mighty pristine force, underlying all organic and inorganic matter. The Yoga which treats of this Kundalini-Sakti is called Kundalini-Yoga.[35]

Kundalini is the Divine Cosmic Energy in bodies. Siddhi or perfection in Yoga is achieved by arousing this Supreme Force which is lying dormant in the Muladhara Chakra at the base of the spinal column in the form of a serpent with 3 1/2 coils. That Yogi in whom the Kundalini is awakened and taken towards the top of the head is the real King of kings or Emperor of emperors. He has all divine powers. All Siddhis and Riddhis (minor powers) roll under his feet. He can command Nature. He can command the five elements. His glory is indescribable.

Before proceeding to know something about the Chakras and the Kundalini-Sakti, it is essential to know something about the spinal column and the Nadis or nerve-currents. The spinal column is called *Meru-danda*,

---

35 *For detailed particulars on the subject vide my book "Kundalini Yoga."*

and it extends from the *Kanda* (situated between the anus and the root of the reproductory organ) to the base of the skull. There are two Nadis on either side of the spinal column called *Ida* and *Pingala*, and between these two runs a hollow canal called *Sushumna* at the lower extremity of which lies the Kundalini-Sakti sleeping a trance-sleep *(Yoga Nidra)*. Ida starts from the right testicle and Pingala from the left, and they both meet the Sushumna at the Muladhara Chakra. Ida flows through the left nostril, and Pingala through the right. Ida is cooling, while Pingala is heating. Sushumna which originates at the Muladhara Chakra runs right up to the top of the head. Ida and Pingala indicate time; Sushumna is the devourer of time. When the Prana flows through the Sushumna, "the most highly beloved of the Yogins", the mind becomes quite steady. The Yogi defies death by devitalising Ida and Pingala and taking the Prana through the Sushumna to the crown of the head or Brahmarandhra (Seat of Brahman). When the Kundalini is awakened, it forces its way through the Sushumna, and its progress is characterised by supernatural visions, acquisition of various special powers, knowledge, peace and bliss. When the Kundalini is taken to the Sahasrara Chakra (at the top of the head). The Yogi enjoys Supreme Bliss.

When the Kundalini enters the Sushumna Nadi, the Prana also enters the Sushumna of itself along with the Kundalini. Regular practice of Uddiyana Bandha awakens the Kundalini and enables it to rise upwards along the Sushumna. This is a powerful Yogic Kriya. All Kundalini enthusiasts should practise this daily. The practice of Yoga-Asanas. Pranayama, Mudras and Bandhas is prescribed only to awaken the Kundalini. These are all potent practices in rousing this great pristine Force.

A detailed knowledge of Nadis (psychic nerves or astral tubes for carrying Prana) and the Chakras (lotuses or psychic nerve-currents) is of paramount importance for all students of Kundalini-Yoga. The psychic nerve lodged in the hollow of the spinal column is the chief or medium Nadi. It is called the Sushumna Nadi. Just as electricity is stored up in dynamos, so also the vital force (Prana) is stored up in the Chakras and the Sushumna Nadi. Prana plays a vital part in all psycho-physical processes. The first attempt on the part of the young Kundalini-Yogi is the purification of the Nadis which will lead to the opening of the Sushumna which generally remains closed up in all worldly-minded people.

All students of Kundalini-Yoga should possess a clear and sound knowledge of the six Chakras. Then only they can contemplate on these Chakras. Meditation on these Chakras brings psychic powers. A Chakra means a centre of spiritual energy. The different plexuses in the human body correspond tentatively to the different Chakras in the astral (Sukshma) body. Otherwise Hatha-Yoga is impossible. There is difference of opinion as to where the Chakras are really located. Doctors dissect the physical body. They are not able to find the centres, lotuses and so forth. Some say that the Chakras are situated only in the astral body. Some others maintain that the Chakras are developed during the course of meditation through the force of Dhyana (contemplation), and that they are not in the astral body. This is the real truth viz., *that the Chakras are in a dormant state in the Pranamaya Kosha (vital air-sheath) of the astral body and that they become opened owing to intense and deep meditation.*

There are six subtle Chakras or centres or lotuses in this Sushumna Nadi. These are *Muladhara, Svadhishthana, Manipura, Anahata, Vishuddha* and *Ajna.* Above all these there is the *Sahasrara,* the chief of all the centres. All the Chakras are intimately connected with the Sahasrara Chakra. Hence it is not included as one among the six Chakras. Sahasrara is situated above all the six Chakras at the top of the head.

The MULADHARA CHAKRA is situated between the root of the reproductory organ and the anus at the base of the

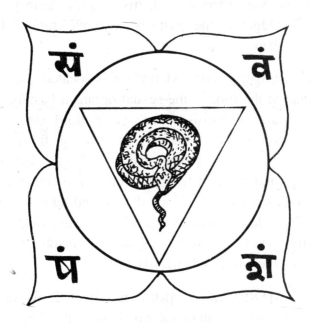

**Muladhara Chakra**

spinal column. It is here, as I have already mentioned, that the two Nadis, Ida and Pingala, meet the Sushumna. The Muladhara Chakra is two fingers above the anus and two fingers below the genitals and four fingers in width. It has four petals of crimson hue. In the pericarp of this Chakra there is a beautiful triangle in which the sleeping Kundalini of the form of a coiled-up serpent dwells. She holds her tail in her mouth and covers the mouth of the Brahma-dvara (the gateway to the Seat of Brahman) with her head. The Yogi who concentrates on the Muladhara Chakra gets full knowledge of the Kundalini and the various means to rouse it to action. As soon as the Kundalini is roused, the Yogi gets the power to rise up above the ground. He gets full control over his breath, mind and semen. His Prana flows through the Sushumna and all his sins are destroyed. He gets knowledge of the past, present and future. He is immensely happy.

The SVADHISHTHANA CHAKRA is located within the Sushumna at the root of the sexual organ. It has six petals and is pure blood-like red (vermilion) in colour. Concentration on this Chakra frees the Yogi from fear of water. He gets several other psychic powers, intuitional knowledge and freedom from the faults of the mind and the senses. He becomes an object of love and adoration to all beautiful goddesses, and recites all the Sastras unknown to him before. He becomes the conqueror of death and moves throughout the universe fearlessly.

The MANIPURA CHAKRA is situated within the Sushumna in the region of the navel and is the third Chakra from the Muladhara. It is of the colour of dark clouds and

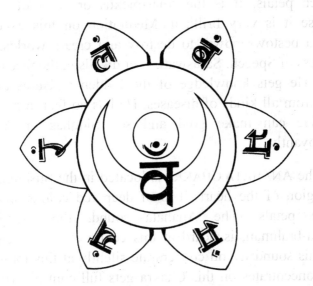

**Svadhishthana Chakra**

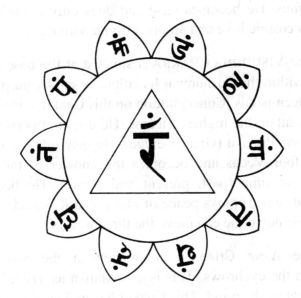

**Manipura Chakra**

has ten petals. It is the solar-plexus or "city of gems" because it is very brilliant. Meditation on this excellent Chakra bestows power to destroy and create worlds. The Goddess of Speech, Saraswati, ever dwells in the face of the Yogi. He gets knowledge of the hidden treasures and is freed from all kinds of diseases. He has no fear at all from fire. He can make gold and see Siddhas or Adepts clairvoyantly.

The ANAHATA CHAKRA is located in the Sushumna in the region of the heart. It is of deep red colour and has twelve petals. The Anahata sound, the sound of Shabda-brahman, is heard at this centre. You can clearly hear this sound if you concentrate silently at this lotus. He who concentrates on this Chakra gets full control over air. He can fly in the air, enter the body of another and become prosperous. He becomes wise and does only noble deeds. He gets cosmic love and all other divine virtues.

The VISUDDHA CHAKRA is situated at the base of the throat within the Sushumna. Its colour is smoky purple and has sixteen petals. Concentration on this Chakra enables the Yogi to attain the highest success. He does not perish even during the Pralaya (Great Deluge). He gets full knowledge of the four Vedas and becomes the knower of the three periods of time (past, present and future). He becomes eloquent, wise, enjoys peace of mind, and it is said that by his Yogic power he can move the three worlds.

The AJNA CHAKRA is situated in the Sushumna between the eyebrows. This is also known as Trikuti. This is the seat of the mind. This Chakra has two petals and is of beautiful white colour. He who concentrates on this most

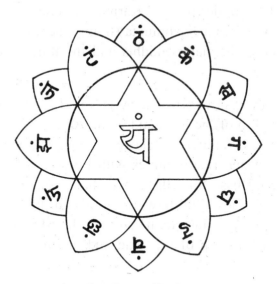

**Anahata Chakra**

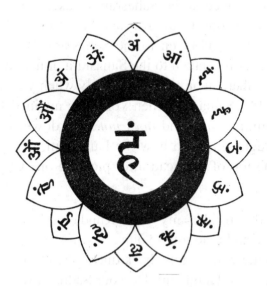

**Visuddha Chakra**

excellent Chakra destroys all Karmas or actions of the past lives and becomes a Jivanmukta (living liberated sage). He gets all the eight major Siddhis and the thirty-two minor Siddhis.

The SAHASRARA CHAKRA is the thousand-petalled lotus at the top of the head and is the Abode of Lord Siva. When the Kundalini is awakened, it pierces one Chakra after another and finally unites with Lord Siva and enjoys the Highest Bliss. Now the Yogi attains super conscious state and becomes a full-blown Jnani. He drinks the Nectar of Immortality. Illustration shows the ascent of the Kundalini to the top of the head and its union with Lord Siva.

When the Kundalini is awakened, it does not directly proceed all at once to the Sahasrara Chakra. You will have to take it from one Chakra to another. You will certainly live even after it is taken to the Sahasrara. But remember that even after it is taken to the Sahasrara, it may drop down to the Muladhara at any moment! Only when you are firmly established in Samadhi, when you have attained Kaivalya, the Kundalini *cannot* and *does not* drop down. Illustration gives a rough idea as to how the Kundalini, when aroused, reaches the top of the head after piercing one Chakra after another.

Do not mistake, my dear Kundalini brothers! O ye enthusiastic and emotional young Yogins! the movement of the rheumatic winds in the back due to the chronic lumbago for the ascent of Kundalini. Do your Sadhana with patience, perseverance, cheerfulness and courage, till you get the Nirvikalpa Samadhi.

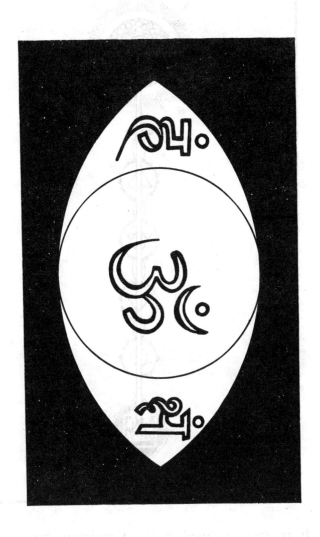

Ajna Chakra

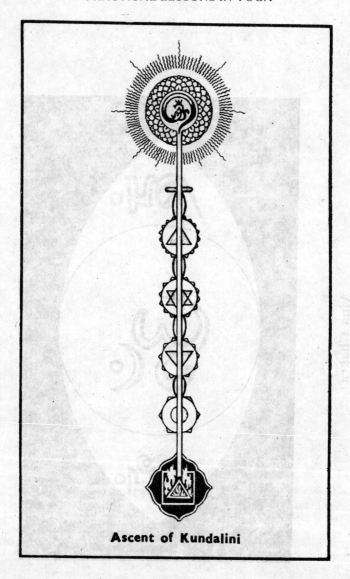

**Ascent of Kundalini**

It is easy to awaken the Kundalini, but it is very difficult to take it up to the navel, to the Ajna Chakra, and thence to the Sahasrara in the head. It demands a great deal of patience and persistence on the part of the practitioner.

But there is nothing impossible for a man of determination and iron-will. That Yogi who has taken the Kundalini to the Sahasrara is the real master of the forces of Nature. Generally Yogic students abandon their Sadhana on account of false satisfaction. They foolishly imagine that they have reached the goal, when they get some mystic experiences and powers. This is a mistake. Complete Asamprajnata Samadhi (Nirvikalpa Samadhi) alone can give final emancipation.

Some Yogic students ask me: "How long should one practise Sirshasana or Paschimottanasana or Kumbhaka or Maha Mudra to awaken the Kundalini? Nothing is mentioned about this point in any treatise on Yoga." A student starts his Sadhana from the point or stage where he left in his previous birth. That is the reason why Lord Krishna says to Arjuna: "Or he may be born in a family of wise Yogins. There he recovereth the characteristics belonging to his former body and with these he again laboureth for perfection. O joy of the Kurus," (Bhagavad-Gita Ch, VI-42, 43).

So it all depends upon the degree of purity, stage of evolution, the amount of purification of the Nadis and the Pranamaya Kosha, and above all the degree of Vairagya and yearning for liberation.

Develop virtues like generosity, forgiveness and so forth. Mere Yogic Kriyas alone will not help you much. Do self-analysis and eradicate your faults and evil habits. Rectify your defects like selfishness, pride, jealousy, hatred, etc. Develop your heart. Share what you have with others. Do selfless service. Then alone you will get purity of mind.

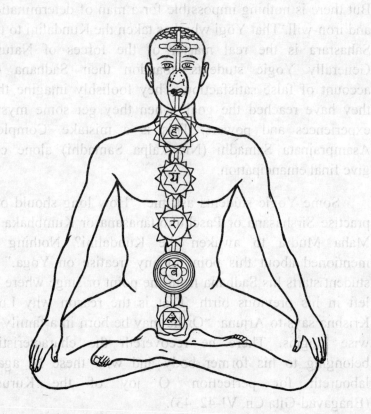

## Shat-Chakras, Ida, Pingala, and Sushumna Nadis

In these days aspirants neglect these things and jump at once to do Yogic Kriyas for getting Siddhis. It is a serious Himalayan blunder. They have the hopeless downfall sooner or later. Therefore be careful. Mere Yogic Kriyas cannot bring in much results. Purification of the heart is very necessary. Without it no success in Yoga is possible. You should free yourself from lust, anger, greed, jealousy, hatred, egoism, vanity, attachment, delusion, etc. This is more difficult than the control of the heart or the practice of Nauli or the uniting of Prana and Apana.

Kundalini can be awakened by various methods such as Japa; devotion, Vichara (enquiry of "Who am I"), Asana. Kumbhaka, Bandhas, Mudras, and above all by the Grace of the Guru. You must become perfectly desireless and free from all earthly longings.

Many persons jump with curiosity and expectation of acquiring occult powers and rousing the Kundalini. They do Sirshasana and various other Asanas and Pranayama. But no one sticks to the practice for a sufficient length of time. They leave off the practice after a few months. This is not good. Application and tenacity, patience and perseverance are essential for sure success and acquisition of Siddhis.

My advice is: Never care for Siddhis or quick awakening of the Kundalini. Have devotion to God. Have perfect trust in Him. Have the spirit of service to humanity. The Kundalini will awaken by itself.

Awakening of Kundalini is not so easy as you may imagine. It is extremely difficult. When all desires die out, when the mind becomes absolutely pure, when all the senses are subdued, when you attain one-pointedness of mind to a considerable degree, when all the ideas of egoism and "mine-ness" melt away, the Kundalini will awaken by itself. Then alone awakening of the Kundalini is also beneficial. Therefore purify yourself first. Have full trust and faith in the Mother. She will do the needful for you at the proper time.

Be not troubled. Be not anxious, my dear friends and brothers! A glorious day is waiting to dawn on you. You will shine with full powers, nay, you will become God Himself. Laugh at all troubles and obstacles and keep your eye on the Kundalini-Sakti all the twenty-four hours. Do all you can in order to rouse her up. If purification is ordained, purify you must. What other alternative is there? Therefore do purify yourself.

O Mother Kundalini! Having pierced the six Chakras, Thou sportest with Thy consort Paramasiva in the thousand-petalled lotus of the Sahasrara Chakra all alone! Salutations unto Thee! Guide me. Give me Light and Knowledge!

# SPIRITUAL VIBRATIONS AND AURA

Vibration means motion. The Lord willed and there was a vibration. The world was projected. The sound OM emanated. The three qualities viz., Sattva, Rajas and Tamas differentiated themselves from the unmanifested. There was a vibration in the ether and the other four elements came forth. Through the process of quintuplication or mixing up of the elements the phenomenal world came into being.

The whole universe is full of molecular vibrations. Any word or Mantra uttered silently or forcibly produces molecular waves, gross, subtle, or more subtle. These waves spread throughout the universe. It is said that the radiowaves move round the world seven times a second.

Everything in this world, both visible and invisible, constantly vibrates. All particles of matter are in a state of vibration. From the tiniest atom to the mightiest planet all things are in a state of vibration. The atoms of the human body are in constant vibration. Different rates of vibration balanced in the cosmic rhythm produce, before us the magnanimous world. Matter is being acted upon by energy and innumerable forms are produced. Forms break down incessantly and new forms come into being. There is nothing in absolute rest in nature. The air is ever vibrating. Rivers are ever flowing. The earth is ever revolving. The stars are ever moving. Forms come and go but the reality that lies behind these forms is unchangeable.

Earthquakes, landslides, volcanic eruptions, thunder, lightning and so forth, are the outcome of vibration. Electricity and magnetism are vibrations only. Music is vibration. If various kinds of musical instruments are kept in a room, properly tuned, and if one instrument is kept in vibration, all other instruments also will vibrate themselves. Music produces harmonious vibrations in the mind and soothes the nerves and the mind.

Every thought, every word and every physical action produces a molecular vibration in the atmosphere which affect every object. Any evil thought, evil word or evil action immediately creates a bad vibration in the atmosphere and does harm to many persons. Conversely any good thought, good word or good action immediately produces a good vibration and does good to many persons.

Telepathy is thought-vibration. The mind is constantly vibrating. The mind is acted upon by the psychic Prana or subtle energy and various thoughtforms are produced. Thought vibrates. The trained Yogi can send a thought in the ether to any distance he likes. Thoughts are separated from each other by different rates of vibration. Wherever and whenever any work is done, a motion or vibration is caused; wherever and whenever a motion or vibration is produced, a sound is produced. The sound of the first motion of the equipoised Nature in the act of creation of Pranava or OM. The Lord willed at the end of the dissolution (Maha-Pralaya): "May I become many." There arose a motion or vibration in the unmanifested Nature (Prakriti). It is Omkara or Pranava-Nada.

There must be harmony or concord in vibration. Then there is peace. There must be rhythm in vibration. Then there is order. There is rhythm in the systolic and diastolic movements of the heart during contraction and dilation. So there is order in internal harmony in the circulation of blood. Man enjoys good health. There is rhythm in the vibration or the movement of the lungs. So man is hale and hearty. If there is a disturbance of the rhythm in the motion of either the heart or the lungs, then man gets incurable diseases of the heart and the lungs and passes away soon.

Some vibrations can be felt or detected by ordinary physical and sensory means. When you shake hands with another man, a distinct vibration can be felt passing from one hand to the other. A man who is both blind and deaf can easily know one individual from another because no two persons have the same vibrations.

You will observe a definite rhythm in all vibrations. The law of rhythm operates in the working of this human machine. There is rhythm in every movement in this universe. Inhalation and exhalation, the systole and diastole of the heart, the ebb tide and the flood tide in the sea, the movements of the stars and the planets in the firmament, days and nights, seasons and monsoons—all follow definite rhythmic laws.

Everything has a different rate of vibration. Various sorts of waves are passing about in this universe. Some waves oppose each other and bring about discord, disharmony and rupture. Some other waves move harmoniously side by side. Then there is peace and harmony. You must know how to harmonise your physical and mental vibrations with those without. Then only you can be really happy. If you can place yourself in tune with the vibrations of another man, you can really understand him. If you have immense liking for another man, it means your vibrations are in tune with the vibrations of that man. People of similar vibrations are united by friendship. If the vibrations of one man strike against those of another, they cannot be united. Hatred, prejudice, dislike and jealousy will result.

The five sheaths[36] should vibrate harmoniously. Then only you will have good health and a sound mind. Disease is nothing but disharmony in the vibrations of the human body. Asanas, Pranayama, recitation of the Names of the Lord, singing hymns and prayer, study of philosophical books will produce harmonious vibrations in the physical, vital, mental, intellectual and blissful sheaths respectively. Then only you can practise meditation nicely.

Colours have vibrations. Some colours are soothing and pleasing, while others are very annoying and irritating. Green colour is very pleasing. Colours that irritate clash in vibrations with those of the receptive subject.

---

36*The five sheaths of the human body are: Food sheath, Vital sheath, Mental sheath, Intellectual sheath and Blissful sheath. These sheaths have concealed the Atman or God within. You will have to pierce through these five sheaths, if you want to see God face to face.*

The vibrations set up by the pronunciation of the monosyllable OM are so powerful that they would bring the strongest building to the ground, if the pronunciation is persistently repeated in the right way.

A note on the violin, if sounded repeatedly in rhythm, will generate vibrations which will in time destroy a bridge. The vibrations caused by the rhythmic movements of the soldiers on a bridge may bring down the bridge. A Yogi practises rhythmic breathing to absorb Prana and develop will. His whole system vibrates harmoniously. There is perfect harmony in the vibrations of his mind. Through rhythmic breathing he transmits an increased current of Prana or nerve-force to any part of the body for stimulating and invigorating it. He renovates and vivifies the whole system and heals any diseased part by supplying an increased quantity of Prana. He transmits powerful thoughts to others to heal them of their disease and attracts countless persons like a powerful magnet. He becomes a mighty centre of spiritual force.

Why do the places of pilgrimage attract people? Because Saints, Mahatmas, Yogins and Sannyasins had done their Tapas and meditation in these places. In other words, these places have been saturated with pure vibrations. That is the reason why the pilgrims feel inexpressible joy, peace and strength in these places. The powerful spiritual thoughts of those spiritual giants are still floating in the atmosphere. They exercise a benign and soothing influence on their minds. Places like Gangotri, Uttarkasi, Badrinarayan, Manasasarovar, Mount Kailas, Rishikesh, Amarnath; and Kedarnath in India are filled with holy vibrations of sages and Rishis of yore who did severe Tapas there, and are therefore best suited and highly beneficial to aspirants for the practice of meditation. Aspirants can enter into the meditative mood in these places without any effort.

Even some places in the plains have their own good vibrations. So some people feel happy in some localities but not in others. Happy surroundings with harmonious vibrations help a man to turn out good, substantial work, whereas unpleasant surroundings with morbid vibrations retard the work of man.

The elements differ, not in substance, but only in the rate of vibrations. The substance in ice, water, steam and vapour is the same. Each contains two atoms of hydrogen and one atom of oxygen, but the rate of vibration differs in ice, water and steam.

If you are ,not powerful to protect yourself, vicious thoughts of others will affect you, when you live with them in the same room. Create a protective magnetic aura around you. Feel and imagine that a protective shell has been actually formed around your body. Practise Pranayama and meditation regularly. No wrong vibrations from without can affect you. Your body and mind will be proof against undesirable vibrations.

If you have a pure mind, if you are free from prejudice, intolerance, dislike, hatred and greed, if you possess love, sympathy, mercy and unbiased neutral state of consciousness, you will be able to find out at once what sort of vibrations people around you radiate. You will develop a new spiritual sense or Yogic faculty.

Do not be carried away by bubbling emotions. Bring them under your control. Use your reason. Keep a balance between reason and feeling. Develop both the head and the heart. Then only there will be harmonious vibrations inside. Regular meditation will pave a long way in the attainment of the balanced state.

If you live in the company of a developed saint, you will be immensely benefited by his wonderfully powerful spiritual vibrations and aura. Even a rank materialist and a confirmed atheist will feel the presence of God in his company.

Man draws his Prana from the air he breathes, from the food he eats, and from the beverage he drinks. You can imbibe the energy from the solar energy also, if you know the Yogic technique. Deficiency of Prana induces weakness, low vitality, languor and inertia. A sufficient supply of Prana makes a man nimble, active and energetic. He has full life in every limb. He jumps and dances in joy.

The aura is in fact an emanation or radiation of life-force from the vehicles or sheaths of man. The aura can be seen only by the Yogi who has inner Yogic sight or clairvoyant vision. Each sheath radiates its own particular aura with a particular rate of vibration. So there is no interference. The auras of the different sheaths interpenetrate each other.

The aura that emanates from the physical body is gross. This is known as the "Health Aura." Its colour is faintly brilliant viole-tgrey or bluish-white mist. It is almost colourless. It is ovoid in shape. It extends from the body to distance of 2 or 3 feet. The "Health Aura" is striated by countless fine lines which project from the body evenly like stiff bristles. In perfect health these lines are separate and parallel. They are in an orderly manner. In poor health or diseased condition they droop down like the soft hair of an animal or the stems of faded flowers. The lines lie about in all directions in a state of confusion. When a sick person recovers from his illness, the radiation of the magnetic form of vital energy slowly begins and the lines of the "Health Aura" are brought back into order. They again become straight and parallel.

Just as blood flows along arteries and veins, so also the vital force flows along the nerves in a constant stream. This vital force is poured upon us from the sun, which is the source of life. He who has abundant vital force is a healthy man. He radiates abundant "Health Aura" and brings joy, strength, health and vitality to countless persons with whom he comes in contact. He becomes a centre of energy. The vital force constantly radiates from his body in all directions. A mesmeriser actually transmits his vital force through magnetic "passes" to the subject. It is through the help of this vital force that he practises various sorts of healing. He who is endowed with abundant "Health Aura" and vital force cannot succumb easily to any disease. The "Health Aura" and the vital force act as powerful germicides. They prevent the entry of germs into the body. Even if he succumbs to any kind of disease, he will tide over the crisis very easily in a short time on account of his high standard of health and vitality. He will convalesce very quickly.

On the contrary a weak man who is deficient in vital force or Prana absorbs the vitality or Prana of a strong man with whom he happens to come in contact. If you feel weak, uncomfortable and weary after an interview with any weak person, remember that the weak man has depleted your energy to some extent. He has acted the part of a vampire. You might have all experienced this in your daily life.

It is quite possible by an effort of the will to put a check to the radiation of vitality from one's body by building a shell around the body. This will prevent the entry of disease-causing germs into the body. Further the body will also be impervious to any kind of astral elemental influence from without. You may render yourself immune from any form of vampirism. There will not be any leakage of life-force from your body. The depressing influence of the base thoughts of low-minded people will be obviated. You can live quite comfortably with them in the same room.

This is the way to develop a protecting auric shell: Sit at ease. Retain the breath for a half or one minute. Imagine that you are surrounded by a shell of thought-aura to a distance of 2 or 3 feet from the body on all sides. Form a clear mental image. Repeat this process 10 to 15 times. Repeat OM mentally, when you retain the breath.

The spiritual aura is of yellow colour. It centres round the heads of Saints, Sages, Rishis, Prophets, and Yogins.

This can sometimes be seen by ordinary persons with naked eyes, when the saint stands on the pulpit to preach. The yellow glow is intensified, when the intellectual faculties are put to an unusual strain. The face of the saint will present a glowing appearance. This is the nimbus or glory of a saint. This is the halo shown in pictures of spiritual leaders. The magnetic spiritual aura of Lord Buddha extended to a distance of 3 miles all around. Those who came within the compass of 3 miles were subdued. They became his disciples. The magnetic divine aura of Yogi Kaka Bhusunda radiated to a distance of eight miles! The spiritual aura of even a first-class aspirant radiates to a distance of 400 yards. You can also develop this spiritual aura by regular and continued practice of meditation with zeal and persistence.

Human aura has different colours in different people according to their growth and development physically, mentally, morally and spiritually, and each colour has got its own meaning and significance. The meanings of some of these colours are set below:

*Scarlet* represents anger.

*Crimson* represents love.

*Rose* represents love.

*Black* denotes hatred and malice.

*Red* on a black background indicates anger.

*Red* on a green background shows jealousy.

*Red* independent of a background denotes "righteous indignation."

*Lurid Sanguinary Red* indicates sensuality.

*Grey* represents selfishness when the colour is bright.

*Grey* represents fear when its shade is like a dead body.

*Green* denotes jealousy when the colour is dirty.

*Red Flashes* on a green background signifies anger mingled with jealousy.

*Slimy Green* signifies deceit and cunning.

*Green* when bright indicates tolerance, tact, adaptability, politeness and intelligence.

*Orange* when bright denotes pride and ambition.

*Yellow* denotes intellectuality. It is a good colour. When the intellect runs into low channels, the yellow is deep and dull. When it is directed towards higher things, it becomes brilliantly golden or prim-rose yellow.

*Blue* when dark and clear denotes religious feeling. When the blue amounts to a rich violet, it represents highest religious thought and feeling.

*Blue* when light and luminous represents spirituality.

*White* when pure and effulgent represents the Spirit or
Brahman or GOD.

Dear friend! Surround yourself with harmonious vibrations within and without. Regular meditation will help you in attaining this end. Carry with you wherever you may go, vibrations of power, strength, joy, bliss, peace, kindness, love, mercy and sympathy. Absorb all good vibrations. Dispel all discordant vibrations. Learn to absorb the vibrations of great sages of yore which are floating in the etherial space. Be in tune with the vibrations of the living liberated sages. They will all back you up. May the vibrations of peace and joy flow through your eyes, face, tongue, hands, feet and skin! May whoever comes in contact with you feel this! May the Eternal, Immortal Spirit guide you in your attainment of Self-realisation by developing harmonious vibrations! Om Peace! Peace! Peace!

# DAILY ROUTINE FOR ASPIRANTS

## 1. ELEMENTARY COURSE[37]

Meditation . . . . . . . . . . . . . . . . . . . . . . . . . 1 hr.

      Morning . . . . . . . . . . . . . . . ½ hr.

      Evening . . . . . . . . . . . . . . . ½ hr.

Study . . . . . . . . . . . . . . . . . . . . . . . . . . . . 1 hr.

Asanas . . . . . . . . . . . . . . . . . . . . . . . . . . 15 min.

      Sirshasana . . . . . . . . . . 3 min.

      Sarvangasana . . . . . . . . 3 min.

      Matsyasana . . . . . . . . . 2 min.

      Bhujangasana . . . . . . . . 2 min.

      Salabhasana . . . . . . . . . 1 min

      Dhanurasana . . . . . . . . . 1 min

      Uddiyana . . . . . . . . . . . 1 min

      Relaxation . . . . . . . . . . 2 min

---

[37]Aspirants of the Elementary Course should devote at least 31/2 hours daily for Yogic practices. They should get up at 4 a.m. in the morning and sit for meditation for 15 minutes, and should also have another sitting for 15 minutes in the evening. The following books are recommended for study:—

1. Spiritual Lessons (Part I and II). By Swami Sivananda.
2. Practice of Karma-Yoga. By Swami Sivananda.
3. Practice of Bhakti-Yoga. By Swami Sivananda.
4. Sure Ways for Success in Life and God-realisation. By Swami
                                    Sivananda.
5. Yoga in Daily Life. By Swami Sivananda.
6. Bhagavad-Gita. By A. Mahadeva Sastri (Theosophical Publishing
                                    House, Madras)

Pranayama . . . . . . . . . . . . . . . . . . . . . . . 15 min.

    Puraka-Kumbhaka-Rechaka .  10 min.

    Bhastrika  . . . . . . . . . . 2 min.

    Sitali . . . . . . . . . . . . . 2 min.

    Relaxation . . . . . . . . . . 1 min.

Selfless Service[38]  . . . . . . . . . . . . . . . . . . . . 1 hr.

              Total time....................$3\frac{1}{2}$ hrs.

## 2 INTERMEDIATE COURSE[39]

Meditation . . . . . . . . . . . . . . . . . . . . . . . . . 2 hrs.

    Morning . . . . . . . . . . . . . . 1 hr.

    Evening . . . . . . . . . . . . . 1 hr.

Study . . . . . . . . . . . . . . . . . . . . . . . . . . . . 2 hrs.

Asanas  . . . . . . . . . . . . . . . . . . . . . . . . . $\frac{1}{2}$ hr.

    Sirshasana . . . . . . . . . . 5 min.

    Sarvangasana  . . . . . . . . 5 min.

---

38 Selfless Service consists in serving Society, country and humanity with Atma-Bhava, without the idea of agency, and without expectation of fruits of action. All works are selfless, when done in the right spirit, with a view to help others.

39 Intermediate Course aspirants should devote at least 6 hours daily for Yogic Sadhana. The following are the books specially recommended for their study:
1. Practice of Yoga. By Swami Sivananda Sarasvati.
2. Raja-Yoga (Theory and Practice). By Sivananda Sarasvati.3. Sure Ways for Success in Life and God-realisation. By Swami Sivananda Sarasvati.
4. Dialogues from Upanishads. By Swami Sivananda Sarasvati.
5. Practice of Karma-Yoga. By Swami Sivananda Sarasvati.
6. Practice of Bhakti Yoga. By Swami Sivananda Saraswati.
7. Mind, Its Mysteries and Control. By Swami Sivananda Sarasvati.
8. Bhagavad-Gita. By A. Mahadeva Sastri (Theosophical Publishing House, Madras).
9. Vedanta in Daily Life. By Swami Sivananda Sarasvati

Matsyasana . . . . . . . . . . 3 min.

Bhujangasana . . . . . . . . . 3 min.

Salabhasana . . . . . . . . . 2 min.

Dhanurasana . . . . . . . . . 2 min.

Mayurasana . . . . . . . . . 2 min.

Paschimottanasana . . . . . 3 min.

Uddiyana . . . . . . . . . . 2 min.

Nauli . . . . . . . . . . . . 1 min.

Relaxation . . . . . . . . . 2 min.

Pranayama . . . . . . . . . . . . . . . . . . . . . ½ hr.

Puraka-Kumbhaka- Rechaka    20 min.

Kapalabhati . . . . . . . . . 2 min.

Sitali . . . . . . . . . . . 3 min.

Bhastrika . . . . . . . . . 3 min.

Relaxation . . . . . . . . . 2 min.

Selfless Service . . . . . . . . . . . . . . . . . . . 1 hr.

Total time...............6 hrs.

### 3. ADVANCED COURSE[40]

Meditation . . . . . . . . . . . . . . . . . . . . . . . 6 hrs.

----

[40]Advanced Yogic students should devote 13 1/2 hours purely for solid spiritual Sadhana. They should read the following books and master them thoroughly.

1. Principal Upanishads—Vol. I and II. By Swami Sivananda Sarasvati.
2. Brahma Sutras—Vol. I and II. By Swami Sivananda Sarasvati.
3. Bhagavad-Gita. By A. Mahadeva Sastri (Theosophical Publishing House, Madras).
4. Ten Classical Upanishads. (Published by G.A. Natesan Co., Madras.)
5. Yoga-Vasishtha. By Vihari Lala Mitra. (Taraporewala Sons & Co., Bombay.)
6. Vedanta-Sutras. Translated by George Thibaut. (Taraporewala Sons & Co., Bombay.)
7. Indian Philosophy. By Dr. S. Radhakrishnan. (Taraporewala Sons & Co., Bombay.)

Morning . . . . . . . . . . . . .2 hrs.
Evening . . . . . . . . . . . . 2 hrs.
Night . . . . . . . . . . . . . .2 hrs.
Study . . . . . . . . . . . . . . . . . . . . . . . . 3 hrs.
Asanas . . . . . . . . . . . . . . . . . . . . . . . . ½ hr.

Sirshasana . . . . . . . . . . 3 min.
Sarvangasana . . . . . . . . 3 min.
Matsyasana . . . . . . . . . 3 min.
Bhujangasana . . . . . . . . 3 min.
Salabhasana . . . . . . . . . 3 min.
Dhanurasana . . . . . . . . . 3 min.
Mayurasana . . . . . . . . . 3 min.
Paschimottanasana . . . . . 3 min.
Uddiyana . . . . . . . . . . 3 min.
Nauli . . . . . . . . . . . . 3 min.

Pranayama . . . . . . . . . . . . . . . . . . . . . . 1 hr.

Puraka-Kumbhaka-Rechaka . 45 min.
Kapalabhati . . . . . . . . . 3 min.
Sitali . . . . . . . . . . . . . 3 min.
Sitkari . . . . . . . . . . . . 3 min.
Bhastrika . . . . . . . . . . 3 min.
Relaxation . . . . . . . . . . 3 min.

Selfless Service . . . . . . . . . . . . . . . . . . . 3 hrs.

Total time . . . . . . . . . . . . . 13½ hrs.

## HOW TO MAINTAIN A SPIRITUAL DIARY

Every one of you should maintain a Spiritual Diary. The importance of a Spiritual Diary cannot be overestimated. Those students who are already in the habit of doing so, know its incalculable advantages. A Spiritual

8. Brihadaranyaka Upanishad. By Swami Madhavananda (Advaita Ashram, Mayavati, Almora.)
9. Mandukya Upanishad. By Manilal N. Trivedi. (Theosophical Publishing House, Adayar, Madras.)

Diary is a whip, as it were, to goad you on towards God. The Diary is therefore your teacher and guide. If you wish to grow spiritually and morally, if you wish to evolve more rapidly, keep a daily record of all your actions.

All great men of the world keep diaries. The life of Benjamin Franklin is known to you all. He kept a daily diary. He noted down the number of untruths and wrong actions for which he was directly or indirectly responsible during the course of the day and endeavoured to rid himself of those faults. By doing so he became a perfect man in course of time. He had full and perfect control over his mind.

You should note down in your Diary the answers to the several questions set forth in the foregoing table after having done or fulfilled the particular thing expected of you. You should turn over the pages of your Diary once in a week. If you can maintain a record of your actions every hour, need I say that your progress will be even more rapid? You will develop your will and will in time be free from all defects and vices.

The diary helps you to rectify your mistakes then and there. You will know the value of time. Calculate the number of hours you spent for each and every item at the end of every month. You should not utter any falsehood in recording your daily actions. You should, on the contrary, realise that the Diary is meant for your own growth and advancement. You should realise that it is the Diary of a spiritual aspirant treading the path of truth to realise Truth. You should accept your faults boldly and frankly and should endeavour to get rid of them. You should compare the progress of your Sadhana of the present week with that of the previous week. If you are unable to do this, do it at least once in a month. Then you will be in a position to make the various adjustments in the various items and increase the period of meditation and decrease the hours of sleep. Blessed are those who maintain Spiritual Diaries for they shall realise God quickly.

# THE SPIRITUAL DIARY (Weekly)

The Spiritual Diary is a whip for goading the mind towards righteousness and God. If you regularly maintain this diary you will get solace, peace of mind and make quick progress in the spiritual path. Maintain a daily diary and realise the marvellous results.

| No. | Questions | Week 1 | 2 | 3 | 4 | 5 | 6 | 7 | Total |
|---|---|---|---|---|---|---|---|---|---|
| 1. | When did you get up from bed? | | | | | | | | |
| 2. | How many hours did you sleep? | | | | | | | | |
| 3. | How many Malas of Japa? | | | | | | | | |
| 4. | How long in Kirtan? | | | | | | | | |
| 5. | How many Pranayamas? | | | | | | | | |
| 6. | How long did you perform Asanas? | | | | | | | | |
| 7. | How long did you meditate in one Asana? | | | | | | | | |
| 8. | How many Gita Slokas did you read or get by heart? | | | | | | | | |
| 9. | How long in the company of the wise (Satsanga)? | | | | | | | | |
| 10. | How many hours did you observe Mouna? | | | | | | | | |
| 11. | How long in disinterested selfless service? | | | | | | | | |
| 12. | How much did you give in charity? | | | | | | | | |
| 13. | How many Mantras you wrote? | | | | | | | | |
| 14. | How long did you practise physical exercise? | | | | | | | | |
| 15. | How many lies did you tell and with what self-punishment? | | | | | | | | |
| 16. | How many times and how long of anger and with what self-punishment? | | | | | | | | |
| 17. | How many hours you spent in useless company? | | | | | | | | |
| 18. | How many times you failed in Brahmacharya? | | | | | | | | |
| 19. | How long in study of religious books? | | | | | | | | |
| 20. | How many times you failed in the control of evil habits and with what self-punishment? | | | | | | | | |
| 21. | How long you concentrated on your Ishta-Devata (Saguna or Nirguna Dhyana)? | | | | | | | | |
| 22. | How many days did you observe fast and vigil? | | | | | | | | |
| 23. | Were you regular in your meditation? | | | | | | | | |
| 24. | What virtue are you developing? | | | | | | | | |
| 25. | What evil quality are you trying to eradicate? | | | | | | | | |
| 26. | Which Indriya is troubling you most? | | | | | | | | |
| 27. | When did you go to bed? | | | | | | | | |

*Name:*

*Address:*

Signature

# YOGA AND SCIENCE

YOGA and Science are inseparable. Science and Religion are inseparable. Science is part of Religion. Science and Religion are necessary correlatives. Scientists are also monists in one sense. They also emphatically declare that there is only one thing viz., Matter or energy. A Yogi tries to control the mental forces, a scientist the physical forces. This is all the difference between a Yogi and a scientist. A scientist is also an unconscious Raja-Yogi, but his mind works in external grooves.

Before the invention of watch, Yogins used to calculate time by measuring the shadow in day and by the study of the movement of the stars in the heavens at night. They were perfectly exact in their calculations. Astronomy and medicine received their first impulse from the exigencies of religious worship. Yogins have a sound practical knowledge of Ayurveda. One who endeavours to qualify himself as his own doctor can become a Yogi. He has to live sometimes in the jungles and has to treat himself first, whenever diseases manifest. Otherwise his Sadhana will suffer and he cannot have rapid progress in Yoga. You will find in the books on Ayurveda: "A healthy body is a good instrument for doing virtuous actions and practising Yoga." Those who wrote these Ayurvedic books were great Rishis and Yogins.

Science is partially unified knowledge. A scientist observes the laws of Nature, experiments in his laboratory, investigates, infers and draws exact conclusions from his observations. He understands Nature. But he knows nothing of the origin or destiny of Nature! Who made the sun and gave power to its rays? Who combined four parts of nitrogen with one part of oxygen? Who gave power to electrons? Who gave power to atoms to combine into molecules? Who or what made and bestowed upon the ultimate particles of matter their marvellous power of varied interaction? Science does not know this great mystery. On the contrary, Yoga is completely unified knowledge. A Yogi gets inner divine realisation. He clearly sees with his inner Yogic eyes the subtle rudiments of matter. He identifies himself with the Supreme Being who is the Lord of the Prakriti (matter). He gets control over the five elements. He clearly understands the whole mystery of creation through direct intuitional knowledge. The scientist lacks this sort of knowledge. He has only experimental knowledge.

In the matter of evidence in psychological question, the sense-perceptions with which science naturally deals are only second-rate criteria and therefore to be received with caution. The closing of the external channels of sensation is usually the signal for the opening of the psychic, and from all evidence it would seem that the psychic sense is more extensive, acute and in every way more dependable than the physical.

The business of science is generalisation of phenomena; it is the function of philosophy and Yoga to explain. Religion is the practical aspect of philosophy. Philosophy is the rational aspect of religion. The scientist tries to answer the "How" of the problem; the philosopher and the Yogi the "Why" of it. It is a mistake to say that such and such an event occurs because of certain laws of Nature. The laws of Nature do not give any real explanation of the phenomena. It is simply a statement in terms as general as possible of what happens under given circumstances in his expression of an observed order or uniformity in a natural phenomena. Science is concerned only with the phenomena. It shows a marvellous harmony of Nature. But it is the problem of philosophy and Yoga to solve the "Why" of Nature's harmony.

Scientists possess partial knowledge of the universe. They have not understood the whole code of Nature's laws. They have no knowledge of the occult side of things. They have no knowledge of the astral, mental and higher planes such as Brahma-Loka (world of Brahma). The unseen world is of far greater importance than the sense-universe which is visible to the naked eye. A fully developed Yogi can function in all the planes and so he has full knowledge of the manifested and unmanifested Nature. The senses by which you get knowledge of the external objects are not fully developed. Therefore the knowledge obtained is partial. The external senses are exact counterparts of the internal astral senses. Scientists have no knowledge of the subtle rudiments of matter. Life will become fuller and richer, when one develops this inner eye-sight by the practice of Yoga. Just as blood, when seen under the microscope, reveals many mysterious things such as leucocytes, lymphocytes, nuclei, pigment, germs, bacilli, etc., so also the inner Yogic eye reveals many mysteries of the hidden side of things. The knowledge of the scientists is only fragmentary or partial whereas the knowledge of the Yogi is full and perfect.

Science differs radically in its outlook from philosophical musings. Consequently the mode of approach to its specific problems is different from that of philosophy. Yet there is some similarity in their findings, when some broad questions are discussed.

Scientists have to learn many things from the Seers of the East. Who gave power to the electrons to revolve? Who gave life to the cell or the protoplasm? What is that power that unites atoms to, from molecules? Who gave intelligence to the cells to secrete milk or bile or gastric juice from the blood? Scientists are still observing and experimenting. They are still groping in darkness. What is the cause of the origin of an impulse? Who is the director of the mind? What is the cause of the origin of thought? Even if all the living scientists were to put their heads together to solve these questions, they cannot give definite conclusive answers.

English-educated people are unduly carried away by scientific theories and discoveries. Anything, however stupid it may be, when stamped by the seal of science, is regarded as gospel of truth. A theory or doctrine, however fallacious it may be, is accepted as true wisdom for all ages, when it is proclaimed in the name and on the authority of science. Even if some fantastic and ludicrous statements are made with the stamp of science by a Haeckel, Einstein or Tyndel, people are quite ready to swallow it with great avidity. Such is the fashion of the day! They reject as base superstition the sublime teachings of the ancient Rishis and Sages. The brains of these so-called educated and cultured people need a prompt, drastic and thorough flushing for a protracted length of time. The poison has percolated into their very cells and tissues.

But I do not mean to condemn the wonderful discoveries and inventions that modern science has contributed to the vast store of knowledge and happiness which the present generation enjoys today. The radio, the aeroplane, the microphone and other marvels of science are bound to baffle human intelligence. Scientists have found ways to fertilise an ovum with chemicals, without the help of semen. It is stupendous success. Some children are also born. They inject the semen that is obtained from renowned and cultured men of the world in order to improve the race. They are attempting to fix a radio in a match-stick. They are trying to get the necessary nutrition to the body by pressing an electric button, so that eating and defecation may be entirely abandoned. They are endeavouring to make the streets move so that there will be no necessity for motor-cars and carriages. They are trying to establish means of communication with the planet Mars. They *may* succeed in all their attempts. May God bless them with roaring success in all their undertakings! But the question is: Can all these comforts and scientific discoveries and inventions give immortality, eternal satisfaction and everlasting peace? Have these material comforts enhanced human happiness? Is not man more restless today than ever before? Is he not more dissatisfied and discontented despite all these comforts? Life has become more complex and intricate. Luxuries are increasing day by day. Even a rich man finds it difficult to make both ends meet. There is only one remedy for all these ills. You will have to abandon all luxuries and go back to simple natural living, if you want to enjoy real and lasting happiness. Immortality can be attained by realising the Self through simple living, practice of Yoga, self-control, mental discipline and meditation.

Matter exists in different conditions or states viz., solid, liquid and gaseous. The conditions may be made to change by variation of pressure and temperature. Water is turned into ice at a low temperature and steam at a higher temperature. Every solid may become a liquid or gas under suitable conditions; every liquid may be rendered solid or gaseous; every gas may be made liquid or solid. One form of energy can be also transmuted into another form of energy. Heat can be transmuted into light and light into electricity. Even so, seminal energy or muscular energy, anger, etc., can be transmuted into spiritual energy (Ojas-Shakti).

There is life in the mineral kingdom. This has been conclusively proved by the experiments of Prof. Van Schron at Naples. Even the elements manifest distinct preference. One element has a strong liking for the company of another. One element may even give up the company of one substance in order to join another element. This is chemical affinity. Every chemist fully knows this well. Hydrogen likes the company of oxygen. Two molecules of hydrogen combine with one molecule of oxygen. Water is formed. If you place sodium in the water, you will notice that oxygen likes sodium better than hydrogen and immediately abandons the company of hydrogen and joins sodium.

Likes and dislikes are more markedly present in the vegetable kingdom than in the mineral. Many plants exhibit a remarkable degree of ingenuity in accomplishing their ends.

You should not think that the different planes or realms are Iying one above another like the trunks in a shop. The different planes fill up the same space and interpenetrate one another like the light of a hurricane lamp, electric light, gas lamp and an ordinary kerosene chimney in a room. Matter has different degrees of density and different planes are constituted according to the different degrees of density of matter. These different planes are not separated in space. You are surrounded by these planes. You can be in touch with these planes, if you develop the inner astral eye or the clairvoyant sight. It is not necessary for you to travel in space to study the condition of these planes. Within the space of the room you have the seven planes interpenetrating each other. The beings of a higher plane cannot be seen by the beings of a lower plane. But a being of the higher plane can see the beings of the lower plane.

According to the theory of Relativity some scientists believe that the world will expand after some years and man of future generations will be seven inches tall only, because matter will have to accommodate now to the increased size of the universe. Some matter is taken out of the bodies of human beings and distributed elsewhere to adjust the state of affairs. This is only a speculation and guesswork of some adventurous scientists. It may not happen at all. So you need not be afraid in the least. Be bold and cheerful. Try to get liberation in this very birth so that there will not be any chance for you to get a tiny body of the size mentioned above even if such an event were to occur. One question strikes me very prominently: Can there be the police department then? Can there be military and naval forces and world-wars? How can a tiny man wield a machine gun? So there will be no world-wars. There will be perfect peace everywhere. Scientists will also have to close down their laboratories. No more inventions and discoveries. No more radios and aeroplanes. No more dictators and tyrants. No more Hitlers and Mussolinis. But Yogins there will always be. Yogins can maintain their usual size. They can even expand their bodies *ad infinitum* through their Mahima Siddhi. They can change their atoms and molecules and rearrange them. They can create new minds, new bodies by their Yogic powers. Even during the Cosmic Deluge they can live. Yogi Kaka Bhusunda lived during many deluges. The position of Yogins is always safe. Yoga is the Supreme Divine Science. It is the Science of sciences. There will be more peace through simple living. Let us pray to have that new happy era soon.

God is the greatest Mathematician. All scientists and astronomers are stunned. They bow down their heads and say: "We cannot proceed further. There is something beyond intellect. Our knowledge is imperfect. The riddle of the universe can be solved only by knowledge of the Greatest Mathematician through intuition. The intellect is a frail and finite instrument. The deductions from various theories have not given us perfect illumination. We are still groping in darkness. We are open to correction. Salutations and adorations to that Greatest Mathematician! Salutations to the Lord of the Universe! May He soon open our inner eyes of intuition!"

He who dwells within this electron or atom, who is within this electron or atom, whose body this electron or atom is, whom this electron or atom does not know, who rules the electron or atom from within is thy Self, Inner Ruler, Immortal. It is this Science of Yoga that can help man to unfold his latent divinity and realise his inner Self, the basis or source of this world, body, mind, electron, atom and all sciences. Let us all pray to the Lord of the Universe and practise Yoga in right earnest and commune with the Lord and obtain Immortality, Supreme Peace and Infinite Bliss!

Om Peace! Peace! Peace!

# GLOSSARY

ABHYASA—Spiritual practice

AHAM BRAHMA ASMI—I am Brahman

ATMAN—The Self

AVIDYA—Nescience

BANDHA—exercise in Hatha Yoga

BHUMA—the Infinite; the unconditioned; Brahman

BINDU—point; seed

BRAHMAMUHURTA—auspicious time between 4 to 6 a.m.

CHAITA NYA—Pure consciousness

CHAKRA—Centre of spiritual energy

CHITTA—Subconscious mind

DHARANA—Concentration

DHYANA—Meditation

EKAGRATA—One-pointedness of mind

GUNA—Quality

ISVARA—Lord, God

JADA—Insentient; non-intelligent

JAPA—Repetition of the Name of the Lord

JIVANMUKTI—Liberation in this life

KAIVALYA—Final emancipation

KAMANDAL—The holy vessel used by a Sannyasin for
keeping water

KARMA—Action operating through the Law of Cause and
Effect

KIRTAN—Singing the Lord's Names

KRIYA—Hatha Yogic exercise

KUNDALINI—The primordial cosmic energy located in the
individual

LAKSHYA—Goal

MAYA—The illusory power of Brahman

MOKSHA—Liberation

MUDRA—A type of exercise in Hatha Yoga

NADA—A mystic sound

NADIS—Nerve-currents

NIRGUNA—Without attributes

NIRVANA—Liberation

NIRVIKALPA—Without the modifications of the mind

OMKARA—The sacred syllable Om symbolising Brahman

PRAKRITI—Nature, the primitive non-intelligent principle

PRANAVA—Same as Om

PRATYAHARA—Abstraction or withdrawal of the senses from their objects

SABDA BRAHMAN—sound-form of Brahman

SAGUNA—With attributes

SAMADHI—The state of superconsciousness where Absoluteness is experienced

SAMSKARA—Impression in the subconscious mind

SATCHIDANANDA—Existence Absolute—Knowledge Absolute—Bliss Absolute; Brahman

SAVIKALPA—With modifications

SOHAM—A Vedantic assertion meaning "I am He (Brahman)"

TAPAS—Penance

TAT TVAM ASI—That Thou Art

TATTVA—Principle, Reality

TRIKUTI—Space between the eyebrows

VEDANTA—(Lit.) End of the Vedas; the school of thought based primarily on the Vedic Upanishads

VIRAT—Macrocosm; the Lord in His form as the manifest universe

VRITTI—A wave of thought, a modification of the mind

YOGA— (Lit. ) Union; union of the individual soul with the
Supreme Soul; any course which makes for such union